How to
Survive Clinical

**ADVICE FROM THE NURSING STUDENTS
AND TEACHERS WHO HAVE BEEN THERE**

Diann L. Martin, PhD, RN

OWENS COMMUNITY COLLEGE
P.O. Box 10,000
Toledo, OH 43699-1947

PUBLISHING

New York

This publication is designed to provide accurate and authoritative information in regard to the subject matter covered. It is sold with the understanding that the publisher is not engaged in rendering legal, accounting, or other professional service. If legal advice or other expert assistance is required, the services of a competent professional should be sought.

© 2008 Kaplan, Inc.

Published by Kaplan Publishing, a division of Kaplan, Inc.
1 Liberty Plaza, 24th Floor
New York, NY 10006

Printed in the United States of America

Library of Congress Cataloging-in-Publication Data

Martin, Diann L.
   How to survive clinical : advice from the nursing students and teachers who have been there / Diann L. Martin.
      p. ; cm.
   ISBN 978-1-4277-9822-0
   1. Nursing--Study and teaching. 2. Clinical competence. 3. Nursing students. 4. Nursing--Vocational guidance. I. Title.
   [DNLM: 1. Nursing Process. 2. Nursing Care. 3. Nursing. 4. Students, Nursing. WY 100 M379h 2008]
   RT71.M33 2008
   610.73071'1--dc22

                              2008029445

10 9 8 7 6 5 4 3 2 1
ISBN-13: 978-1-4277-9822-0

Kaplan Publishing books are available at special quantity discounts to use for sales promotions, employee premiums, or educational purposes. Please email our Special Sales Department to order or for more information at kaplanpublishing@kaplan.com, or write to Kaplan Publishing, 1 Liberty Plaza, 24th Floor, New York, NY 10006.

Contents

About Diann Martin

Dr. Diann L. Martin, former Dean of Nursing at Kaplan University, received her BSN from Loyola University in Chicago in 1974. Both her MSN and PhD are from Rush University in Chicago. Her clinical practice includes 28 years in home health and hospice in which she held a variety of clinical administrative positions. She has also been a health-care consultant, author, and lecturer. She lives in Wilmette, Illinois, with her family and loves being a nurse.

Introduction

My warmest welcome and heartiest congratulations to you as you enter into the profession of nursing. Nurses make up the largest professional talent pool in health care and our national need for nurses is critical. Please take pride in being a student nurse, as your work will make a vital contribution to individual patients and to communities over the span of your career. Remember always that *nurses change lives*. The experiences you have as a student nurse will also change your life and your outlook and perspective on health and illness. You will touch those you care for, and you will be touched forever by your patients.

This book was written *for* student nurses *by* student nurses, along with experienced nurses and nurse educators, to give you practical ideas and strategies for working in your initial clinical rotations. By now you have likely completed much of your general education course work and you have knowledge of the basics of human anatomy and perhaps even pathophysiology. It is time to move closer to the day that the initials *RN* appear after your name by starting your clinical experiences. While clinical experience is exciting and it is what you have been preparing for, it is likely to be anxiety provoking or even downright frightening! These feelings are normal and you will soon gain confidence in your level of knowledge and skill in providing patient care.

I have been a nurse now for over 34 years. My decision to become a nurse was as important and valuable to me as the day I walked on the unit for my first clinical experience. I have witnessed tremendous change and evolution in the delivery of patient care over the course of my career. Nurses today are faced with demands of an increasingly complex technological environment for health-care delivery. They must be smart, compassionate, efficient, and effective. Nurses must help patients achieve the optimal outcomes of care while recognizing the cost of the resources needed to render that care. My wish for you is that you be challenged to think and to learn, not only from your textbooks and your faculty, but from your patients. May this experience find you doing important work. I hope this survival book stimulates your thinking.

Diann L. Martin, PhD, RN

CHAPTER 1

Welcome to Your First Clinical Rotation

STARTING OFF ON THE RIGHT FOOT AND GETTING READY FOR CLINICAL

"I wish someone had told me to breathe."

—Boulder Creek, California; Nursing Student

The greatest gift that you can provide to your patients is your self-confidence and caring. You have prepared yourself for this day; you have been a successful student to this point or you would not be here. You have practiced with fellow students. You have worked in the clinical lab, and you know what you need to do. Nurses who are successful *know* a lot about normal and abnormal body functions, they know how to *do* a lot of technical procedures, and they *care* a lot about their patients and their professional role as nurses.

At this point your best strategy is to focus on observation and assessment. Watch, listen, smell, and feel as you move into the clinical unit. A suggestion (as you are likely to be nervous) is to just stop for a moment. Take in and slowly release a deep breath. Focus on the present moment. High-performing athletes and actors do this prior to a performance. This suggestion deals with the student comment at the opening of the chapter. Conscious breathing is a lesson from meditation and it works! You need to focus and be in the present moment with your patient. To that patient you are the care-giving professional and your caring and competent attitude will go a long way toward inspiring confidence—even on your first day of clinical.

Hospital units are busy and bustling environments. You will see many different health-care staff seemingly in their own worlds, scurrying to address a multitude of patient care needs. It is likely that your senses will be overloaded, so be deliberate in paying attention, taking in information, and knowing what is expected of you in your first clinical assignment. Even if you have worked in a health-care setting, you are likely to feel like a fish out of water in a new and often hectic environment.

Remember that the first rule of nursing is to do no harm. Ask questions if you don't know something. Be polite and kind. Look and act like a professional. Call other health-care team members and patients by their names. Be as prepared as you can be to take care of your patient or complete your assignment. This is a first step on what will hopefully be a long and rewarding career path for you. Make it a memorable step.

The remarks and advice in this chapter are excellent reference points to keep in mind as you begin your first experiences as a nurse. Read them over, think about what is expected of you, and go be a great nurse!

YOU'RE NOT EXPECTED TO KNOW IT ALL

The mark of the educated person is to know what she knows and know what she doesn't know. *None of us know it all.* Part of the role of the learner is to seek input and ask questions. Use your preceptors and your clinical instructor to help and support you.

" • *If you mess up, fess up!*
 • *It is always okay not to know something. It is never okay to pretend you do if you don't.*

- *You have to be willing to be uncomfortable for a while before you get comfortable. (These were the best words of advice ever spoken to me by my own clinical instructor.)*

- *If you don't look dumb in front of someone every day, you probably aren't trying hard enough.*

- *I do not expect you to remember how to do all the things you did in the skills lab step by step or all the pathophysiology you studied in class off the top of your head. Just because I said it doesn't mean you learned it.*

- *If you hide from me, I can't help you.*

- *Remember that almost everything you do will be criticized. This is not to make you feel bad; it is to help you get better.*

- *Come to clinical with an attitude of openness and be willing to learn whatever anyone is willing to teach you.*

- *Speak up!*

- *Make sure you are prepared for clinical each day, including getting some sleep the night before. You will have a much better experience and it will decrease your stress exponentially.*"

—**Dallas, Texas;** Nursing Instructor

KAPLAN

"Take a deep breath. Your teacher will not let you kill your patient."

—**Louisville, Kentucky;** Nursing Student

"You will see and experience things which you would never imagine. You may be overwhelmed by your feelings. If you feel overwhelmed, stop and take a deep breath and center yourself. Ask questions. I am more afraid of a student who knows all the answers."

—**New York, New York;** Nursing Instructor

"I wish someone would have told me how useless I would feel. As a new nursing student, I found myself completely floored by how little I could do, how in the way I felt, and how badly I wanted to help the nurses on the floor. If someone had said, 'Hey, you're going to feel in the way, it's natural,' I would have felt better."

—**Waukegan, Illinois;** Nursing Student

"Everyone feels clueless! No one expects you to know it all; that's why it's called learning!"

—Hanover, Pennsylvania; Nursing Student

"Don't be afraid. Things may seem hard at first, but things are easier once you relax and realize you know the material. If you didn't, you wouldn't be in the position to care for a patient."

—Willingboro, New Jersey; Nursing Student

"Do not expect to know all the answers. However, you should learn how to recognize an information need that you or your patient may have, and where to go to answer that information need."

—New York, New York; Nursing Instructor

"Be patient with yourself as you gain confidence with your skills in nursing school."

—Philadelphia, Pennsylvania; Nursing Instructor

ALWAYS KEEP IN MIND THAT IT'S ALL ABOUT THE PATIENTS

Nurses change lives. From the vantage point of your first clinical rotation, that may seem remote or ethereal but it is true. For example, it is likely that the first pair of eyes that gazed into yours when your mother gave birth to you were those of a nurse; and when the time comes, the last eyes looking into yours may well be those of a nurse. The focus of our profession is the well-being of our patients. As a student, your assignment is usually to care for one or two patients during your clinical hours. Hospitalized patients feel vulnerable and depend on the support and attention from their nursing team. Look beyond the patient's diagnosis, tests, and treatments to the *person*, and be present in the moment with them.

"Never forget the reason you went into nursing. We are all here because we care about people and want to make a difference in their lives. Sometimes the greatest thing we can do has nothing to do with our training and everything to do with our own humanity. Perhaps the patient simply needs someone to listen to them or just hold their hand."

—**Lubbock, Texas;** Nursing Instructor

"Don't make it look like it was the first day on the floor. Your patients don't really want to hear that."

—**Isanti, Minnesota;** Nursing Student

"Your job is to keep your patients safe. Anything short of that is unacceptable."

—**Champaign, Illinois;** Nursing Instructor

"*As corny as this sounds, these are my best words of wisdom: Always remember that your patients are strangers to you and you to them. They are letting you into their lives, with no choice, during some of the most anxiety producing, unsettling, alone times of their lives. They are letting you touch them in intimate ways, help them, hurt them . . . never forget what an extreme privilege and responsibility we have been given.*"

—**Rochester, Minnesota;** Nursing Instructor

CLINICAL IS YOUR OPPORTUNITY TO LEARN

Nursing is an applied science and as such, your student experience is your chance to apply all that you are learning to the care of your patients in the clinical courses. Learning means uncovering information, collecting data, assessing the patient, and providing care. If the elements of care are new and unfamiliar, someone with more experience is there to guide and observe you.

"*Every experience is a learning experience; take advantage of the time you have to learn as much as you can.*"

—**Hayesville, Kansas;** Nursing Student

"*Relax and don't try to be a 'super nurse' the first day. Use this time to learn how to put your skills in action.*"

—**Atlanta, Georgia;** Nursing Instructor

"*Take advantage of every opportunity to perform a skill.*"

—**La Porte, Texas;** Nursing Student

"*It is important to work on your assertiveness. You are more likely to get invited into experiences if you ask and seek out opportunities and obviously want to learn. Don't just sit back and wait for someone to come get you or take you with them to an experience.*"

—**Bakersfield, California;** Nursing Instructor

"Take even the simplest tasks very seriously and perfect them to the best of your ability."

   —Boston, Massachusetts; Nursing Student

"You have to be the one to obtain the knowledge you need. Do not rely on your preceptor."

   —Glendale, Arizona; Nursing Student

"Don't be afraid to jump right in. Clinical instructors like that about new nurses."

   —Tracy, California; Nursing Student

"Before you start clinical, review basic nursing skills. If possible, find out what kind of unit you will be assigned to so you can review the types of diagnoses you'll be working with."

   —Philadelphia, Pennsylvania; Nursing Instructor

CLINICAL WON'T BE EASY, BUT THAT'S OKAY!

Nursing is not for sissies. Nurses work hard physically and mentally. Sometimes, due to illness, fatigue, or discomfort, patients are not able to show you their gratitude. They may in fact display behavior that is hostile or critical. Keep in mind that this is NOT about you—it is about them and their anxiety. You need to know that most patients are grateful for your attention and caring. Clinical experiences will stretch you at times, maybe wear you out at times, but they will prepare you for the transition from being a novice to an expert.

"No matter how stupid you feel, every nurse in the building was once in your shoes. Also, having the right attitude will go a long way in how your patient perceives care and how your coworkers perceive whether or not you are a team player. None of us is a hero working alone. Learning to accept your own deficits and to work toward minimizing them is a step toward personal fulfillment. Nursing is hard work. Do not expect otherwise. Nursing can be very rewarding. Embrace change. Without change there would be *no butterflies. You cannot take care of others if you do not learn to care for yourself.*"

—**Longview, Texas;** Nursing Instructor

"*I wish someone would have told me that you will feel like quitting many times and that it's totally normal to feel that way, but it's all worth it in the end.*"

—**San Antonio, Texas;** Nursing Student

"*You will make mistakes and be nervous, but you will gain your own style and technique. Trust in yourself!*"

—**Eau Claire, Wisconsin;** Nursing Student

"*Don't be afraid of the stereotypical 'mean nurse'; there are lots of nurses who love to help students learn.*"

—**Greenville, South Carolina;** Nursing Student

"I wish someone would have told me how intimidating it can be. Even more so, how important it is to be confident in front of the patient."

—Abilene, Texas; Nursing Student

"Be proud of your status of nurse. Define it and wear it with humility and confidence."

—Brookeland, Texas; Nursing Instructor

Nurses change lives. You have decided to change yours by seeking a career as a professional nurse. Right now you are in the learning mode. As a learner you will be shown the way and guided in your experience. If you do not feel that you have been given the resources, support, or supervision you need to do your best, speak up in a professional and honest way with your faculty or preceptor. Take the time after each clinical experience to reflect on what you saw, what you did, and how your patient responded. Apply the nursing process model to your day on the unit:

- **Assessment:** What did you see and feel on the patient care unit today? What was happening? What was happening with your patient today?

- **Observations:** What data did you collect or monitor? What signs and symptoms of disease or illness did your patient display? What was his/her functional status?

- **Interventions:** What care did you provide to your patient—not only physically, but emotionally? Did you provide any patient teaching?

- **Evaluation:** How did the day go? For your patient? For you? Is there anything you feel that you could have done to improve or learn for the next experience?

Nursing is an important and intimate trust between you, the patient, and other members of the health-care team. Give yourself the freedom to be a learner. Your responsibility as a student is to be prepared, seek guidance when you need it, and to *let your caring show.*

CHAPTER 2

How to Remain Organized in a Sea of Information

WHAT METHODS WILL BEST PREPARE YOU FOR CLINICAL?

" Organization is the keystone upon which everything else rests. If you are not organized, you cannot effectively and safely take care of patients."

—Iowa City, Iowa; Nursing Instructor

Developing and maintaining solid organizational skills will be a key to your professional success as a nurse. It is no surprise that many people who are attracted to nursing have a personality type that prefers order and systematic thinking. If you are one of these types, great—you may already be ahead of the game. If you are not, you are going to have to learn some new habits and integrate them into your routine . . . at least professionally. Organizing is best when it is comprehensive and multifaceted. Think about your time, your materials, key data and information, and your energy expenditure in performing patient care.

Organized people live by some simple and basic rules. They plan their work, and then work their plans. As a nursing student, you will likely be given your patient assignment or clinical activity expectations in advance. This information is your opportunity to do some prework and preparation before you hit the clinical unit. In earlier times, this was called patient care planning. Hopefully you will have the chance to read and learn about your patient's medical problem, age, and some other basic demographics. Use any information you are given to identify the potential nursing needs your patient could present with. The challenges that impact preplanning may include shorter inpatient stays, last minute changes in clinical patient care assignments, and the bombardment of too much information to digest in a short time span.

When you are in the clinical setting, you will be more efficient and effective if you take the time to organize and prepare your patient care materials and supplies. Try to avoid being in the midst of a patient care procedure and needing to leave to go to the utility room for the tape or bandage that you forgot. You also want to avoid multiple treks down the hospital corridors if you can. Likewise, find a way to organize information—both reference information that you will need and the pieces of information and data that you collect. This data storage and retrieval system could be anything from a small spiral notebook in your pocket to a handheld PDA. The idea here is to find a system that works for you and use it as you proceed through your day.

Last, give some thought to conserving energy, both your patients' and your own. Most sick people tire easily. Think about ways to optimize their energy, such as coordinating a time for them to sit in a bedside chair while you change their bed linen or having them put on a fresh gown while you help them up to the bathroom. You will learn more tricks of the trade as you observe other nurses and nursing assistants in the clinical setting.

WORKING OUTSIDE OF THE HOSPITAL

So you are getting ready to provide patient care. Until you have some experience under your belt, you will need to do some studying and maybe get some practice in the skills lab to be ready and well prepared. Read your textbook and look up information about the patient's medications if you have a list handy. Does the patient's age or ethnic or cultural background have any bearing on the care you will need to provide? Here are some helpful suggestions that others have offered.

"*Read before class. This sounds silly, but it's amazing how few students actually do this. Don't blame your instructors for what you don't learn. Turn off the TV.*"

—**Fort Gibson, Oklahoma;** Nursing Instructor

"*Research patient history, diagnosis, medications, and disease processes the night before.*"

—**Atlanta, Georgia;** Nursing Student

"*Every student needs to know his or herself—do you put things off until the last minute, or do you go home the first day of class and outline the entire textbook? I was very unorganized clinically (I had pieces of paper in all my pockets), but that system worked for me. Now I would probably encourage my student not to do that, but if it works . . .*

I stress that students need to find at least one half hour each night to review what was presented in class; this gives them a chance to see what they understand and what is unclear. The same with clinical: think about the day and write down what went well and what could be changed the next time."

—Old Bridge, New Jersey; Nursing Instructor

"*I always worked ahead. By reading ahead, it enabled me to retain more knowledge. While this is difficult to do with the large amount of reading, I learned more by reading what we were going to be discussing.*"

—West Bend, Wisconsin; Nursing Student

KAPLAN

"*I stayed in my office until my work was done and ready for the next day. That way I had no distractions.*"

—**Lewisville, Texas;** Nursing Student

"*The lack of preparation prior to the clinical experience is certainly one of the most common errors made by nursing students. Students need to devote quality time to preparing for their upcoming clinical day. They need to research everything they can about the patient's disease process, treatment, and prognosis. Additionally, students must be aware of all prescribed medications the patient is receiving . . . including the classification, mechanism of action, dosage, patient teaching, and adverse effects.*"

—**Jacksonville, Florida;** Nursing Instructor

"*I used my textbooks and pharmacology book to prepare for my clinical assignments. With an understanding of the disease process and the ordered medications, I was able to organize and prepare for my patient(s).*"

—**McHenry, Illinois;** Nursing Student

"Always do your homework the night before. Keep a one-page medication chart of each patient's meds for quick reference. Note cards are great to have, but they can be time-consuming for finding each med when your instructor is reviewing."

—**Pasadena, California;** Nursing Student

DON'T LEAVE IT UP TO MEMORY

We live in the information age and much of the facts and data that we need to recall can be stored in devices that literally fit into the palms of our hands. You may want to look into the purchase of a handheld data device or PDA (personal data assistant) that allows you to store and retrieve vital information about medications, signs and symptoms, diseases, or laboratory test information. Make sure you have an available way to record patient information in *real* time so that you can complete an accurate and timely patient record.

"Carry a small notebook with you at all times!"

—**Madison, Indiana;** Nursing Instructor

KAPLAN

"*Write everything down. There is so much going on that if you don't write everything down, even the small stuff, important information can get lost in the tide of information coming at you.*"

—**Minneapolis, Minnesota;** Nursing Student

"*Individual folders or notebooks for each clinical or class worked well for me, as well as a calendar with all assignment and test dates so that I could see what the priority was at the moment.*"

—**Charleston, South Carolina;** Nursing Instructor

"*I wrote everything down because it gets really overwhelming at first. I always thought I had to do everything really fast, when in fact I was left with nothing to do after I got everything done. Take your time!*"

—**Houston, Texas;** Nursing Student

"*Color coding is a time-honored method among nurses to stay organized—color code your notebooks for each course. Keep everything for your courses—you may be able to use something either when you graduate or in another course. Don't get behind. Study every day.*"

—**Lincoln, Nebraska;** Nursing Instructor

"*Don't cram. Nursing school is a process, not a race. There is so much information to digest, so when cramming, you will suffer unless you are blessed with a fantastic memory.*"

—**Owasso, Oklahoma;** Nursing Student

"*I use a 'box' system. Anything I know that I need to do, assess, teach, etc., I write down and put a box next to it. Once it's done, I 'x' it out. This keeps me on track. I've shared this with students, and many of them love it.*"

—**Manalapan, New Jersey;** Nursing Instructor

"*I used a three-ring binder with tabs categorizing each section, with a special section for resources/handouts that would be useful when I needed information quickly. I used my computer to keep a medication bank with an index that I updated with each new medication. I made sure to know what equipment was being used for each patient (such as T-tubes, peg tubes, etc.) and looked up or asked their nurse what the purpose was for each. Knowing the purpose of treatments and medications prepares you for an easier and more successful clinical day.*"

—**North Aurora, Illinois;** Nursing Student

"*I like to write everything down. That way it is right there for you to look back on without having to use up precious time trying to find the information again in the chart. Find it once, write it down once, look at it anytime you want!*"

—**Minneapolis, Minnesota;** Nursing Student

PREPARATION STARTS BEFORE YOUR CLINICALS

Clinical experiences and the logistics of how the work is organized and assigned will vary from school to school and from one clinical experience to the next. The major takeaway theme is that you need to use whatever tools and resources you have been given or can locate to be as knowledgeable and prepared for your patient care experience as you can be.

"
- *Always come prepared—meaning know your drugs, lab values, diagnoses, etc.*
- *Come to the clinical setting with two plans in mind. That way you will have a backup plan should the first one fall through (always keeping in mind that you are dealing with people, and even the second plan may fall through).*
- *If the PIXES is busy, don't stand around waiting—go do something else, then come back.*
- *Document as you go; don't leave it until the end of the shift.*"

—Mechanicsville, Maryland; Nursing Instructor

" *Most preparation was done by going to the hospital/facility the night before, getting the patient's chart to whom I was assigned, and looking up the pertinent data needed for appropriate nursing care to be given. I also carried my PDA with me, which contained a drug reference guide, lab guide, medical dictionary, etc. I carried it with me in my pocket the day of clinical just in case I needed to make a quick reference. I also tried to carry my textbook pertaining to that particular clinical with me and/or used another person's text for reference. I also carried a clipboard to organize my paperwork, with a small chart on the front of it that detailed my actions for the day broken into hourly increments (e.g., 8 A.M.: give patient bath and substitute medications).* "

—**Baltimore, Maryland; Nursing Student**

" *When in clinical, I tell my students to make hourly goals. What do you want to accomplish by 9 A.M. to stay on track? If you find that you are behind schedule, how can you get back to where you need to be? It really makes the students think about what is important.*

In theory courses, students need to make a study calendar so that they can keep up with the reading. Whenever something doesn't make sense, go to someone and figure it out! Don't wait until the last minute before an exam to try to find a faculty member. Last, make sure that you plan time for yourself! Having designated times on the calendar for fun really helps decrease the stress."

—La Plata, Maryland; Nursing Instructor

"*I always like to plan ahead of time and anticipate that there is always something new to learn every day. That way, even if it doesn't go the way I expected it to, I can still be able to put up with the situation and certain unexpected assignments that come my way.*"

—Mesa, Arizona; Nursing Student

KAPLAN

MAKE YOUR LIFE AS EASY AS POSSIBLE

Think of yourself on the clinical unit as if you were in a time-and-motion study. What pieces of equipment will you need to take care of your patient? Where are the supplies located? How can you use your time most wisely by being prepared in advance? Do you have all of the requisite items in the same place *before* you need them? Having said this, do not become a pack rat or take *all* of the clean towels in the patient's room. Just try to think through what materials and equipment you and the patient will need. The drill here is reminiscent of the TV handyman show *This Old House,* where you are told to "measure twice and cut once."

"*Take that extra moment to organize your stuff, and you will be so much better off.*"

—Louisville, Kentucky; Nursing Instructor

"*I was at clinical earlier than I had to be. I had my backpack set down, my clipboard ready. I made sure the BP machine I was going to use was where I wanted it to be. I stocked my med cart at that time with cotton balls, 4 x 4s, etc. When we were allowed to get report, I received my patient, printed out my MARs, and checked the cardex and chart. I noticed that when my classmates arrived on the floor right on time, they would go set down their backpacks, get supplies, and by that time I already had my vitals on my patients.*"

—**Bakersfield, California;** Nursing Student

"*If you have small children, look for high school students in your area that can come in for several hours in the late afternoon or evening to give you time to study. The money spent will be well worth it.*"

—**Mishawaka, Indiana;** Nursing Instructor

" • *Keep all school supplies—books, notes, assign-ments—in a specific place at home and make that area off limits to others in the household.*

• *Get a notebook/folder for each separate nursing class.*

- *Carry a loose-leaf notebook with tabbed dividers for each class and as soon as handouts are given, three-hole punch them, and put them in the notebook under the proper tab.*

- *Leave room in your classroom notes for additions that you might want to make after reading more about the subject or after looking up unknown words.*

- *Organize your backpack/book bag for the next day before you go to bed at night.*

- *Get a planner of some type, either hard copy or electronic, and plot out everything on it, including available study time.*

- *Post a calendar on the refrigerator with the schedule of everyone in the house, so all can see when people are available and when they are not and so everyone can see how the household has to work together, instead of mom being responsible for everything.*"

—Kansas City, Missouri; Nursing Instructor

"*Don't wait until the last minute to do papers and projects. When you rush through things, it shows and will affect your grade.*"

—Union Beach, New Jersey; Nursing Instructor

"Identify what is 'need to do' versus 'nice to do.' Study every day even if only for a short period of time. Get help when needed, not when you are failing."

—**Cypress, Texas;** Nursing Instructor

USE YOUR INSTRUCTORS AND YOUR PEERS

Major resources for you in the clinical area are other experts and your peers. The unit staff nurses generally enjoy helping students learn the ropes and will give you ideas and suggestions. Your instructor is available to you to do just that—*instruct*. If you find yourself with an extra few moments, ask a fellow student or a staff nurse if you can observe or assist with a patient procedure. It will also be helpful to work together as you provide some aspects of patient care. You may have a large patient, or someone with very limited mobility. The buddy system can be a manageable way to learn together and to accomplish more together than you may have been able to do solo.

"Try to learn one new organizational skill from a nurse on staff and then master it in your clinical assignment each week."

—Bayville, New Jersey; Nursing Student

"Find a 'buddy' in your classes and clinicals. Procrastination is a deadly sin in nursing school. Friends and 'study buddies' will help to keep you on track. There is a tendency to try to team up with someone on the same level you are—resist it. Try to get into the 'overachievers' study group. You will get better grades and be more likely to stay on top of assignments."

—Pueblo, Colorado; Nursing Instructor

"*Getting behind in nursing school can be almost disastrous. Take accountability for your own learning, but know that other students are in your same situation. Study groups help many students, especially in exam preparation. In one school in which I taught, the students would establish study groups and divide the objectives for a given exam. Each student would carefully prepare the information appropriate to his/her assigned objectives, and then the group would share the information with each other. It worked very well for them.*"

—Southside, Alabama; Nursing Instructor

Nursing practice and your clinical experiences will challenge you to be organized and efficient in conducting your work. These skills evolve and sharpen over time, so give yourself a chance and you will improve incrementally. To summarize, you can help your patients and be more effective if you get and stay organized. Prepare for clinical care in advance. Find tools and techniques to store and retrieve patient information readily. And finally, your most valuable resources are the other nurses and your fellow students, who can help and support your learning.

CHAPTER 3

Coordinating the Theory Class with Your Clinical Rotation

INSTRUCTORS OFFER TIPS ON HOW TO BRIDGE THE DIVIDE

> "Recognize that theory is a necessary part of the training; however, focus on the patient care and look at every patient as a person and not as a theory."
>
> —**Centennial, Colorado;** Nursing Instructor

In considering nursing education, you will often hear the term *theory* as opposed to *clinical* learning. The point here is that you will be involved in both classroom learning and in applying what you have learned to the clinical setting. Sometimes by design and by good luck, the two types of learning will come together into a nice, neat whole. But sometimes they may be out of sync. Through no fault of your clinical instructors, the clinical setting and its realities may not provide you with an exact and timely fit between what you are studying in class and what types of patients you will be assigned to in clinical practice. Shortened lengths of inpatient hospital stays and increasing use of ambulatory practice mean that student experiences will be less of an obvious fit with classroom instruction. It may be up to you, the student, to tie the pieces together and extrapolate to make the clinical experience a rich and rewarding one. Let's consider an example to make this clearer.

In class this week you are studying cardiovascular illness with a focus on heart disease. You review normal circulation and the impact of illnesses such as heart attack and congestive heart failure. You learn about anticoagulant medications, beta-blockers, and how the impact of poor circulation and profusion affects the patient's energy. You then go to clinical and get assigned to a stroke patient. Well—all is not lost. Your patient has had a cerebral vascular insult and compromised circulation to the brain. Likely some tissue death occurred, so use your critical thinking skills to figure out how this vascular insult is similar to loss of blood flow to the heart muscle. What functional losses is your patient experiencing? What is the patient's energy level? What nursing needs are manifesting in relation to the cerebral vascular accident? It is likely that you will still need to help this patient recover and that the care you provide will be restorative in nature. You should be able to apply concepts and principles of care that you learned about in class.

Clinical and classroom instructors should be working together to help support your learning. The content you are learning should be conceptual and broad enough to apply across a variety of types of patients and their disease states. For example, any patient who has limited mobility will need to have care that attends to their skin integrity, bowel and bladder function, nutritional status, and hygiene. Clinical faculty can best support students in their clinical settings by using prototypic sample cases that require you to apply general concepts from theory to actual patient scenarios. In preclinical and postclinical conferences, they can bring up discussion questions or patient care problems that highlight or review the material covered in class. Many nursing concepts, such as patient safety, cut across all age and diagnostic groups. In this chapter, instructors draw on their experience to share unique ideas about how to tie classroom and practice together.

"*Think before you go to clinical about how you can bring what you learned in the classroom to the bedside. After you go home, think about what went well (and why) and what didn't go so well (and why). Keep asking 'why?' until you have an answer. If you draw a mental blank, excuse yourself from the room and go find a quiet place to review what you know and need to know or do. Have notes in your pocket about what you need to do so you can review this. The restroom is sometimes the best place to accomplish this.*"

—St. Paul, Minnesota; Nursing Instructor

"*If you are caring for patients with diagnoses you have already studied, go back and review text and class notes. Look over labs and meds and begin to try to understand how this all fits into the big picture.*"

—Florence, Kentucky; Nursing Instructor

"*Ask the questions: What am I seeing and how does that relate to what I read? What should I know to take care of this patient?*"

—**Charlotte Hall, Maryland;** Nursing Instructor

"*Think critically about why you are doing a particular patient care activity. It should always be based on evidence from nursing- and medical-related research.*"

—**New York, New York;** Nursing Instructor

"*Do more than go through the motions. Think about the theory behind what you are doing. Why do you do what you do? Why should you wait and give a bath before a meal or several hours after? Why is your patient demanding or angry? Use theory to get insight into what your patient is going through.*"

—**Charleston, South Carolina;** Nursing Instructor

"*Choose patients who have primary or secondary diagnoses that have been recently studied in class. When students do this, they are able to see the sequel of the disease, the meds that go with it, the associated assessment findings, etc. They get the whole picture and it helps them understand. This sounds basic, but students often choose patients based on the number of meds they get to give or skills they anticipate being able to practice (dressing changes, injections, etc.). Also, if possible, simulated clinical experiences should be used to fill in the gaps for content that has not been reinforced in the hospital.*"

—Dallas, Texas; Nursing Instructor

"*Read the book. Most students don't like to read and try to just study the notes instead of reading and trying to understand the concepts. Try to choose patients with diagnoses you are not familiar with so you can learn about a new disease process or new treatment.*"

—Rock Hill, South Carolina; Nursing Instructor

"Ideally, theory and clinical should be taught in tandem. It is also important that students understand that they may be in OB rotation, but the concepts they learned in medical/surgical nursing still pertain to an OB patient, and so on."

—Salt Lake City, Utah; Nursing Instructor

"Embrace theory as the framework to organize your data collection. Understand what the patient is experiencing, and mobilize the interventions to facilitate coping on physiological, psychological, and emotional as well as cognitive and developmental levels. Theoretical frameworks are simply tools to formulate plans of care and move from individual to family and group nursing scopes."

—Brookeland, Texas; Nursing Instructor

"*It is very simple—refer to the notes, the textbook for the theory, and tap into the faculty knowledge for best coordination. Theory courses should be taught using the nursing process as the basis for the content. All textbooks follow this format. So the application of knowledge to clinical should be easy to do when the student follows the nursing process.*"

—De Pere, Wisconsin; Nursing Instructor

"*The students can best coordinate theory class by thinking of theory as a support to nursing practice. I would advise the student to think of nursing as a science involving people, environment, and a process. I would also stress the importance of the nursing model, which involves a methodology of assessing a patient's individual needs and implementing appropriate patient care.*"

—St. Louis, Missouri; Nursing Instructor

"*Bring your notes to clinical when you have a patient who matches what you are learning in class. This will help you apply what you have learned to practice.*"

—**Atlanta, Georgia;** Nursing Instructor

"*Theory should be a part of everything you do and why you do it. It is important to remember that theory and clinical are not separate entities, but in fact complementary. As nurses, we need to know why we make the decisions we make. Embrace the theories taught, but ultimately you must formulate your own, taking account of your own life experiences, goals, and values.*"

—**Lubbock, Texas;** Nursing Instructor

"*For theory projects/papers, pick something that you can apply to clinical/patients if at all possible.*"

—**Bakersfield, California;** Nursing Instructor

> *"Calendar your theory and clinical schedules. Stay organized. Immediately before and after class and clinical, identify your strengths, weaknesses, and areas of improvement to help you personalize your learning needs—then pull the two together."*

—Durham, North Carolina; Nursing Instructor

Remember as you begin your clinical experiences that nursing is an applied science. You will have a great deal of factual and conceptual learning. Although you may or may not have a hands-on experience with applying this information in your clinical practice, look for connections between the concepts you are learning and how these play out with actual patients that you care for. If you are having trouble making these connections, let your clinical faculty member know and discuss the situation among your fellow students. As time passes and you have more clinical experiences, this will get easier.

CHAPTER 4

Working with Patients

HOW TO MANAGE THE GOOD, THE BAD, AND THE IN-BETWEEN WITH GRACE AND RESPECT

"Be patient with all of your patients."

—Freeman, South Dakota; Nursing Student

The core of nursing is providing care to patients. The relationship between a nurse and a patient requires the nurse to behave professionally and hold patient care and private information in trust. In some ways it is a sacred and special form of intimacy. Most people regard their bodies and bodily functions as a private and very personal realm that others are rarely invited or allowed to enter. In the case of people who are sick or disabled, this intimate territory is opened up to nurses and other caregivers. Often the patient has little to no experience with a stranger touching his body, asking probing personal questions, or handling his body fluids. Be aware and be respectful of the *person* in your care. It may sound preachy, but it truly is an example of a time in your life when you should live the golden rule—do unto others as you would have them do to you. Showing respect, maintaining patient privacy, and communicating clearly and honestly are some of the ways that your behavior will support the caregiving role of a professional nurse. This may sound simple, but in reality it can be a challenge. In this chapter, your peers and some instructors will highlight some important behaviors to keep in mind when providing patient care.

"*The two mistakes I see most:*

1. Breach of confidentiality. Students are so eager to discuss the 'cool' things they saw in clinical that they are not careful to withhold identifying information or to discuss things in a contained environment. I still catch a lot of hallway conversations or discussions about one patient in another patient's room.

2. The patient's right of refusal. Either the student gives up too easily ('My patient with dementia said she didn't want a bath, so I'm not going to give her one') or not easily enough ('He said he didn't want to take the medication, but I told him he had to because it was ordered'). **"**

—**Dallas, Texas;** Nursing Instructor

THE PATIENT/NURSE RELATIONSHIP IS ONE WITH RULES AND EXPECTATIONS

As a nurse you are in a unique relationship with another human being. You are a caregiver and a helping person. You can be friendly . . . but not a friend in the traditional sense. You are involved in intimate actions . . . but you are not an intimate partner. You will have a lot of information and details about your patient, and while performing your duties, you will likely gather even more personal information . . . but it is not proper to share it or discuss it outside of your professional interactions. You are in some ways an authority figure who will direct the activities and actions of your patients . . . but you cannot dismiss their free will or self-determination about their care. It is a good idea to think through the realities of the nurse/patient relationship as you begin your clinical practice.

"*Listen and don't try to guess what they are trying to say to speed up the process.*"

—Douglas, Massachusetts; Nursing Student

"*Sometimes students are so excited about their clinical experiences that they discuss client condition in areas that do not ensure confidentiality—conversing on the elevator, on the shuttle bus, etc. Another right that has been breached is removal of confidential info from the acute care setting. Many institutions have printed material that is easily accessible to students. I have seen this info shoved into backpacks to review at home—a total breach of HIPAA rules!*"

—De Pere, Wisconsin; Nursing Instructor

"*Students and other clinicians do not understand that HIPAA is meant to protect privacy and confidentiality—and not to impede the process of high-quality care and information seeking that may appear to infringe upon privacy concerns.*"

—New York, New York; Nursing Instructor

"*Patients' right to know is their right to know . . . as a nurse you can give out results of a blood test, such as blood sugar, if the patient asks. Also, you must be careful about family members. Just because they are with the patient does not mean the patient wants the family to know what is going on. Always ask the patient if it is okay to speak freely in front of family.*"

—Charleston, South Carolina; Nursing Instructor

"*The patient actually does have the right to expect certain behaviors and attitudes and care from the nurse. Once the nurse accepts responsibility and is willing to be accountable for his/her actions, then the patient and the nurse will be on the same page.*"

—Longview, Texas; Nursing Instructor

"*Students forget about the patient's right to refuse. They are so eager to help, they forget patients can refuse care.*"

—Atlanta, Georgia; Nursing Instructor

"Nursing students should never forget rules of informed consent. Make sure that patients understand what is happening and why it is happening, not just 'because the doctor said so.'"

—Durham, North Carolina; Nursing Instructor

"Students fail to fully comprehend patient confidentiality. They can answer all the subject-related exam questions perfectly; but in practice, they share everything with fellow students, family, and their extended support network."

—Virginia Beach, Virginia; Nursing Instructor

"Privacy is very challenging for new nurses since the school experience involves a great deal of discussion and case analysis."

—Holt, Michigan; Nursing Instructor

"*Bottom line: If someone is not directly involved in that patient's care, you should not be discussing that patient with them.*"

—Philadelphia, Pennsylvania; Nursing Student

"*Be yourself. Show your personality, yet remain professional. Look the part in a uniform that demonstrates you care about your appearance. Be honest—let them know what you do know, and that you'll find out what you do not. Answer questions truthfully and therapeutically. Be safe. Know your own knowledge level and when you need to ask for help, look something up, or review.*"

—Phoenix, Arizona; Nursing Instructor

YOU ARE SPEAKING A LANGUAGE THAT IS HARD TO UNDERSTAND—BE PATIENT

As you have progressed through your early education in nursing, you have learned a new language: lots of long words, weird abbreviations, names you never dreamed of for body parts, diseases, treatments, and tests. Most likely it was like a foreign language to you at the beginning—which should make it easier for you to realize that it will be a foreign language to most patients as well. Unless you are a mechanic, this feeling is similar when you take your car in for repairs and are baffled as the mechanic starts describing the problem and the repairs that are needed! Many patients feel lost, vulnerable, and embarrassed by the information overload they get in a health-care setting. You can be supportive and helpful by providing information, speaking clearly, and asking follow-up questions to ensure that the information was, in fact, received and understood. Just the anxiety of being a patient can cause many people to need simple, clear, and repeated information.

Another critical part of communicating effectively with a patient is to remember the basics. Introduce yourself by name. If there is a way to write down and leave your name with the patient, do so. Let the

patient know how long you will be taking care of
him that day and what activities are planned. Always
address the patient by name—and don't presume to
use her first name unless invited to do so. Avoid (like
the plague) using terms of endearment like "honey" or
"sweetie" when addressing a patient. Let the patient
know *what* you plan to do with him *before* you do it.

" *It is very difficult to allow patients who are*
competent to make decisions that we, as medically
trained personnel, know are dangerous. Our job,
as medically trained personnel, is to completely
and thoroughly explain the risks and benefits of
the recommended treatment. The most important
thing to remember is that we must communicate
on a level that patients can understand. I find
that patients often make poor decisions, even
after a physician has explained everything to
them, because the physician spoke with words
the patients could not understand. There are
many instances when the physician explains the
treatment, he or she leaves the room, and the
patient turns to me with a 'deer in the headlights'
look of bewilderment. It then becomes my job
to 'translate' what was said into words they

understand and also relate what was said to situations or circumstances that are applicable to them, in the world they live in. Ultimately, however, the decision is theirs to make, and we must respect that decision. If we have done an effective job in communicating with patients, then hopefully the decision they make will actually be the one they really want, not one made out of ignorance."

—Lubbock, Texas; Nursing Instructor

"I see new nurses who want to 'convince' patients and families to see things their way—the words may not come out per se, but nurses have no place communicating to patients in an 'if I were you' fashion. We can educate, help explore, offer resources, make referrals, and sit in silence and support during difficult times/decisions, but the patient has the ultimate right to do as she/he feels is right. We want them to be informed, not swayed."

—Rochester, Minnesota; Nursing Instructor

"*Sometimes nurses get too busy and do not listen to what the patient says, and that gets the patient upset. Be a good listener.*"

—Glendale, Arizona; Nursing Student

"*I encourage students to practice AIDET: Acknowledge patient, Introduce yourself, Describe what you are doing or are about to do, set the Expectation (e.g., how long it will take, outcome of procedure, etc.), and Thank the patient.*

I help students develop a script such as the following that allows them to become confident in working with patients:

'Hello Mrs. Smith, my name is Joe. I am a third-year nursing student and I will graduate this semester. I have also worked on a medical/ surgery unit as a nursing assistant for five years. I am going to take your vital signs and then report them to your nurse. I should be finished in ten minutes.

Okay, I have your vital signs. Thank you for letting me be a part of your care today.'

It is also important that students have preplanned for their clinical experience. If they know the patient assignment ahead of time, they should be able to articulate the disease process, current treatments, and their nursing interventions. It will help them build their nursing knowledge base, gain confidence, and build trust with their patients."

—Charleston, South Carolina; Nursing Instructor

"*Introduce yourself to your patients, and let them know what you are doing, when you will be doing it, and why. Talk with your patients, and answer their questions. Make them feel as comfortable as possible. I have seen nurses go into a patient's room and do things, and the patient has no idea who they are or what they are doing. By explaining things in terms that patients can understand, a lot of stress and anxiety can be taken away.*"

—Defiance, Ohio; Nursing Student

"Introduce yourself and look professional. Practice introducing yourself in the mirror at home. Role play this with family. It is important to look confident when you introduce yourself to your client!"

—**Madison, Indiana;** Nursing Instructor

"Become a partner with your patient to formulate their care based on what is important to them. Be sure to educate them about the care and disease process, being sure they understand and know the choices they have and the outcomes of those choices."

—**Denver, Colorado;** Nursing Instructor

YOU'RE NOT IN THIS ALONE

Once again, whether it is your first day in clinical or you have been a nurse for 20 years, you will never have all of the answers. No one will. If a patient asks you something that you do not know (and they definitely will), tell them directly that you do not know but will try to help them find out. You may need to ask a staff member, your instructor, or refer to the chart or a reference book to get additional information. You will realize that some patients hang on every piece of information given to them by a nurse or a doctor. Make sure that you are truly listening to patients and their questions as you communicate.

"*Don't be scared of hurting them. The nurses you will be working with and your instructors are not going to let you.*"

—Cincinnati, Ohio; Nursing Student

"*Don't be afraid to say 'I don't know, but I'll find out for you.'*"

—**Kansas City, Missouri;** Nursing Instructor

"*If a patient asks you questions and you have no idea what the answer is, tell him you will ask the nurse and get back to him. Do not assume you know everything or think you know everything because you do not want to give him false or incorrect information. And trust me, patients will ask questions!*"

—**Ewing, New Jersey;** Nursing Student

"*Seek out experienced nurses and observe how they interact with clients.*"

—**Mount Laurel, New Jersey;** Nursing Instructor

WHEN THE GOING GETS ROUGH, THE ROUGH GET GOING

As a student there will be times when you are in clinical, but your head and heart may not be. Maybe you stayed up too late; maybe you had to study for an exam in another course. You are just not in the Florence Nightingale mood, but there you are anyway. In other words, the situation, the patient's personality, or some other issue is in your way. Times like this call upon nurses to push through the moment, collect their thoughts, and focus on the present. Remember, this is not about *you*, it is about your patient. The patient wants and needs a caring professional. If that can't be you, find a fellow student to come in and be a supportive helper as you provide care. Go drink a glass of water, gather your thoughts, and take some deep breaths. These "off" days happen to all nurses. Don't be hard on yourself.

"*Listen and look like you care. Customer service is half the battle.*"

—**St. Joseph, Missouri;** Nursing Instructor

"*Be confident and friendly even though you may not know a darn thing. A smile will not only ease your tension, but that of the patient as well.*"

—Orange Park, Florida; Nursing Student

"*Don't be afraid! Approach with confidence, even if you don't feel confident. Have someone else go into the room with you the first time if you are really nervous.*"

—Charlotte, North Carolina; Nursing Instructor

"*Don't be afraid. Jump in and get your (gloved) hands dirty—it's the only way that you'll learn. Although nursing has stretched the boundaries of what professional responsibilities are available (admin, informatics, sales, research, etc.), the foundation of nursing is bedside care.*"

—Iowa City, Iowa; Nursing Instructor

"*Carry yourself with the attitude that you know exactly what you are doing, no matter how little you really know. The patient doesn't have any idea of your inexperience, and the false confidence you have now will turn into the real thing as you work toward being a nurse. Treat all of your patients with respect and compassion, and just try to get to know them a little bit, and they will surprise you with how much trust they actually put in you.*"

—**Fairless Hills, Pennsylvania;** Nursing Student

"*Treat them as you would want to be treated if you were lying in that bed.*"

—**New Albany, Indiana;** Nursing Student

DON'T FORGET THAT PATIENTS ARE PEOPLE

Sometime in your nursing career, you will hear a nurse or a doctor refer to a patient as the "gallbladder in 420 bed 2" or that "hot abdomen in 550." Such depersonalization unfortunately comes with the trade unless you work diligently from the beginning to humanize your patients and remember that they are people, just like you. The interesting part of being a nurse is that you will meet a wide and diverse array of people: rich and poor, clean and dirty, smart and dumb, sophisticated and base. There is nothing quite like being in a hospital gown with their rear end exposed to level all humans to their basic materials. And every one of the types of people mentioned above commands the same respect, attention, and caring that you have to give as a nurse. Some patients will be kind and respectful to you in return, others will be more difficult—maybe even crabby and contentious. Being sick and vulnerable does not bring out the best in many folks, so learn not to take unpleasant behavior personally. It is most likely not directed at you, but at the frustration and fear of the situation.

"*Respect the client and his/her family. Wear the ID badge in a place where it is easily seen. Introduce yourself and identify yourself as a nursing student. Tell the client and family how long you will be there and that you will be providing most of their care during that period. Address the client as Mr. or Mrs. or Ms., unless specifically asked by the client to call them by a first name. Certainly you can use first names with children or young adolescents, but address parents with terms of respect. Explain procedures before and during administration. Inform the client of his/her role during the procedure, if appropriate, such as, 'It is important that you are very still while I . . . . ' Offer praise after the procedure, even for adults. We never outgrow our need for affirmation.*"

—Southside, Alabama; Nursing Instructor

"*Show you are interested—make it a point to find out one personal anecdote about the patient or his/ her family during your shift. And always remember that a sincere apology goes a long way.*"

—Pueblo, Colorado; Nursing Instructor

"In many cases patients are just as nervous as you are, but they are willing to give you a chance. Just be open and honest. If you promise to do something for them, follow through."

—**Hughesville, Maryland;** Nursing Student

"Always be empathetic—how would you feel if that were you in that bed? Don't get mad at people for being sick and asking for help—that is what you signed up for. Be honest, have kindness, and never forget the person behind the illness."

—**Union Beach, New Jersey;** Nursing Instructor

"Make sure that you check on your client routinely, even if it is to just go in and say hello."

—**La Plata, Maryland;** Nursing Instructor

"Remember that the patients are sick, tired, and in a place they don't want to be."

—**San Jose, California;** Nursing Student

"*Treat them as unique individuals. Do not treat only by what the book says. Everyone is different.*"

—La Porte, Texas; Nursing Student

"*Don't take your clinical forms into the patient room. Don't tell the patient you need to ask a few questions 'for an assignment' in your clinical course. Don't talk about yourself. Don't tell them about your children, or your broken car, or what you had for dinner last night. Don't take your cell phone to clinical. And if you do . . . don't use it.*

Walk all the way into the patient's room; stand at the bedside to talk to them. Use a normal tone of voice. Think about what you would want (or need) if you were in your patient's position. Ask them what they need. Offer suggestions if they say 'nothing.' Review procedures prior to performing them. Know the clinical facility's policy regarding the procedure you are about to perform. Take a bath, brush your teeth, wash and comb your hair, use deodorant . . . but not cologne. Wear a clean uniform without wrinkles. Minimize jewelry and makeup. Your patient will appreciate this. Be organized and efficient, yet demonstrate a personal, caring attitude."

—**Fort Gibson, Oklahoma;** Nursing Instructor

"*Remember that if they are upset or seem unappreciative, it is usually because they don't feel well. Remember that you make a difference.*"

—**Marion, Iowa;** Nursing Student

"*Know yourself, what your values and beliefs are. You will meet many patients who do not fit in with those values, and that will make you uncomfortable or uncertain. If you can recognize that what you are experiencing is a clash of values, then that will be helpful.*"

—**Mishawaka, Indiana;** Nursing Instructor

"Take the time to get to know your patients so that they can trust you—once they can truly trust you, they will communicate their true needs. Remember that all of your patients are important; they are all someone's family, and they deserve the best care you can give them."

—Rochester, Minnesota; Nursing Student

"Continually dialogue with your patients: about what you are doing, what you know, what you do not know. Let them know why you may not be in to see them for a while, let them know you will find the answer to any question they ask. And always be kind."

—Peoria, Illinois; Nursing Instructor

"You stand between life and death for a patient. No matter how bad a day you have working on the floor, chances are the patient has had a worse one."

—Charleston, South Carolina; Nursing Instructor

"Be firm if needed . . . but not bossy."

    —Palmdale, California; Nursing Student

"Don't promise things you cannot keep."

    —Louisville, Kentucky; Nursing Instructor

"Realize that some patients will not like you. Get over the personal issue and realize that they are not always upset at you."

    —St. Clair Shores, Minnesota; Nursing Student

"Be nonjudgmental, especially when a patient's values or decisions are different than your own."

    —Edmonds, Washington; Nursing Instructor

"No matter how nervous you are, no matter how much you feel you are infringing on their privacy, think about what you would want . . . the best care, right? Well sometimes that means interruptions of sleep and television programs. Just be polite and explain why you are doing what you are doing. They will come around."

—**Stow, Ohio;** Nursing Student

"I see a lot of professionals talking about work/ patients/inappropriate things in front of other patients, like they aren't even there. Remember that even if sedated, they can often still hear what is going on around them."

—**Minneapolis, Minnesota;** Nursing Student

"If you promise a client something, follow through with it. If you forget, go as soon as you remember and apologize to the client and then do what you promised to do."

—**Mechanicsville, Maryland;** Nursing Instructor

YOUR TIME IS PRECIOUS, BUT USE IT WISELY

Years ago, famous nursing leader Luther Christman studied the sociology of nurses. He found that they tended to spend their time in the nursing station versus with patients when free time was available. This reality is disheartening and only you can change it. You will be busy—sometimes even rushed. The trick is to be present in the moment and work efficiently so that each patient you care for feels that you have all the time you need to take care of his or her needs. Pay attention to your own energy expenditure by being organized and ready to provide care, and pay attention to the patient's energy by not overtaxing him or her in the process of care. If you do have a few free moments, think about sitting at the bedside of someone who is without visitors or who seems lonely or frightened.

"*Since the demands of nursing don't allow you to spend inordinate amounts of time with your patients, be present when you are with them.*"

—Denver, Colorado; Nursing Student

"I find after 35 years of nursing and six of teaching that most patients love having students care for them, and I tell my students this. Patients know for at least that one day they will get the spa treatment and lots of TLC."

—Old Bridge, New Jersey; Nursing Instructor

"Be respectful, considerate, and above all honest with high ethics. Learn assessment, and be thorough to prevent problems as opposed to treating complications that could have been prevented. Never get in a rush when administering medications; don't let anyone hurry you up."

—Cypress, Texas; Nursing Instructor

"I spend time talking to my patients. I can find out more in ten minutes than one hour of looking at the chart. I can also tell if something is wrong before the lab tells me. This is because I take the time to get to know them."

—Phoenix, Arizona; Nursing Student

"*Understand that sick people have limited energy. Do not ask questions unless needed. Introduce yourself and your plan of care before you put your hands on the patient. Announce your presence in the room by introducing yourself; this gives the patient time to 'wake up' and realize what is going on. Plan your work to conserve the energy of the patient and yourself. Have all of your supplies, linens, etc. before you begin. Review procedures with your faculty member or nurse before you enter the room.*"

—Lincoln, Nebraska; Nursing Instructor

"*Take your time to ask questions. This gives you a chance to get familiar with patients and identify their concerns.*"

—Los Angeles, California; Nursing Student

Your most gratifying moments of being a nurse will come from the interactions and time you spend with your patients. What you give to others as a nurse will truly come back to you in the gratitude and support from your patients. Working with patients requires that you maintain a professional demeanor, be a good listener, and use your time and attention wisely.

CHAPTER 5

Working with the Health-Care Team

FINDING YOUR PLACE AMONG YOUR NEW COWORKERS

"Communication, communication, communication. Oh, did I say communication?"

—Denver, Colorado; Nursing Instructor

In most patient care situations, both as a student and as a registered nurse, you will be working as part of a team with other health-care providers, along with patients and their families. Each member of the team has a unique but oftentimes overlapping role with you, the nurse. Your job is to reinforce the work of other team members and simultaneously fulfill the nursing needs of the patient. During the course of a hospital stay, for example, a patient may encounter up to 20–30 different health-care providers. No wonder patients are confused and unclear on whom to seek for information and support! As a nurse, you will most often be handling and managing the patient's *response* to illness, disease, and diagnosis. You will help the patient recover or restore his or her capacity to the maximal level possible. You will serve the patient as a provider of care and treatment, a health educator, and an advocate. You will also help interpret the patient's care needs and treatment to other members of the team.

SOMETIMES YOU HAVE TO HAVE A THICK SKIN

The old days of grumpy hierarchical physicians and nurses as handmaidens are for the most part long gone. You will find that physicians value nurses who are competent and caring professionals. In the beginning of your clinical experience, take note of the nurses you observe who have positive interpersonal relationships with other members of the health-care team. What behaviors do they exhibit that earn the trust and esteem of their teammates? When a team member exhibits unprofessional or noncollegial behavior, can you identify what is behind the behavior? Remember that working with sick people can be draining and at times unfulfilling and frustrating. As in direct patient care, you will need to learn not to allow yourself to be the victim of someone else's bad day.

"*Most of your interactions will be good ones, but there will be some people who are not good with students. Seek out the ones who are supportive. I found that there are nurses who nurture you and others who tolerate you. Some nurses have shown me the kind of nurse I do not want to be like. You learn both sides in the clinical setting, and this will help you in the future.*"

—Manchester, Wisconsin; Nursing Student

"*Don't wear your heart on your sleeve. Doctors get upset and sometimes say harsh things when patients are not getting well, equipment doesn't work, or department results are not back in a timely manner. Remain professional and don't take remarks personally.*"

—Phoenix, Arizona; Nursing Instructor

"*Just be patient. Sometimes nurses forget that they were students once upon a time.*"

—Brea, California; Nursing Student

"*Some health-care staff love students and some don't. If you know what's going on with your patients and are prepared to care for them, then you are ready to work with either.*"

—San Jose, California; Nursing Student

"*Some people will be really helpful and nice and some will range from indifferent to mean. Just keep your head up and show them you are a hard worker and you want to learn.*"

—Blanchard, Oklahoma; Nursing Student

"*Remember that the health care team is under stress from the shortage of nurses and the current health care settings. Do not take too much to heart and only accept constructive criticism.*"

—Philadelphia, Pennsylvania; Nursing Instructor

"Don't be alarmed when you get the brush-off from some of the more experienced nurses. Don't let the nurse's aides take advantage of you; remember, you are there to be a nurse, not an aide."

—Austin, Arkansas; Nursing Student

"The health-care team is not there to act like an instructor. They are there to care for patients. Now, I personally do not feel that gives staff an excuse to be rude. Some staff members are more helpful than others; but remember, holding your hand is not their job."

—Norfolk, Nebraska; Nursing Student

"Just know that not every experience is going to be good. However, you can learn from every experience (even if it is just teaching you how not to respond to nursing students!)."

—Saint Cloud, Minnesota; Nursing Student

THE NURSE/STUDENT RELATIONSHIP IS A GIVE-AND-TAKE

A great deal of your learning in clinical practice will come from observing experienced nurses. They will give you lots of tips and show you some valuable and practical ways to manage patient care. The best teachers will neither take over a task as you stand on the sidelines, nor leave you high and dry on your own. They may talk you through a procedure and then watch you perform it, step by step. This type of coaching and support is a great way to build your confidence and to help you learn new skills. Having the chance to work with students is a source of pride for many experienced nurses. Think about it—wouldn't you enjoy having a chance to be an expert? Remember to thank the staff for their help and support. Nurses who work with students generally have to take extra time and attention for this role, and in many settings there is no additional pay or reward for this activity. Let the expert know how much you appreciate his or her time and talent.

"*Remember that you are a learner and a novice. Without being patronizing, acknowledge the staff's knowledge and experience. Usually students are reluctant, especially in new clinical settings, and the attitude of the unit staff in receiving them and welcoming them as learners is crucial. Remember that you are a visitor on their unit. Respect their unit in the same way you would respect a home in which you are visiting. Never forget the value of 'please' and 'thank you.'*

Let it be known that you would like to be included in observing procedures that you have not seen before, but position yourself to not be in the way. Realize that confidentiality may require that you not be present in certain situations. Avoid any unprofessional behavior with other students or with the unit staff (i.e., no flirting). Remember from the moment you walk on the unit until the moment you leave, you are a health-care professional."

—Southside, Alabama; Nursing Instructor

"*There are those who will love to teach you and have you there. Take advantage of those people because there will be those who will not want you there and will treat you like you are from the bottom of the barrel.*"

—Rockford, Illinois; Nursing Student

"*Nurses are busy. Do not expect that they will stop their work to give a detailed explanation to you. However, they will answer your question in a short manner, and they are willing to show how to do procedures and manage equipment.*"

—Bishop, Texas; Nursing Student

"*Collaboration is paramount during rounds. Listen and contribute.*"

—Kings Park, New York; Nursing Instructor

"*I had good experiences, but not everyone did. I feel it is important to be willing to do non-nursing tasks to help the preceptor. The preceptor in return will be more willing to spend time helping you practice new skills.*"

—Turnersville, New Jersey; Nursing Student

"*Arrive on a new unit wanting to learn and listen. Develop relationships whenever you can. Be slow about criticizing on a new unit. Let others help you, ask for help.*"

—Peoria, Illinois; Nursing Instructor

"*My experience was good. I can tell you what I did: I acknowledged the RN as someone I could learn from and thanked her for her time. I was kind and attempted to behave in such a way that they knew I understood that it was a privilege to be there and that I was grateful for the experience. I never had a bad experience, and I believe it was due to my attitude.*"

—Hurst, Texas; Nursing Student

"*Be confident that what you have to contribute is important.*"

—**Mount Laurel, New Jersey;** Nursing Instructor

"*Let the nurse manager know of team members that are student advocates or went the extra mile.*"

—**Greenville, South Carolina;** Nursing Instructor

ACT LIKE YOU WANT TO BE THERE

Remember the earlier discussion about nurses hanging around the nurses' station? Try to avoid this at all costs. If you are finished giving care to your patient, help someone else or go observe another nurse or make rounds on the unit. It is up to you to be self-motivated to get the most out of each day you spend in a clinical setting. If it is a light day, perhaps you can go and observe a diagnostic test or a procedure that one of your patients is scheduled for. Maybe you could update a patient's care plan or help admit a new patient to the unit. You will be getting more out of the experience if you seek these additional activities.

"*Be positive and act glad to be there. Come as a learner, willing to learn new things and be taught. Be professional in dress and mannerisms. Follow the rules. Understand that as a student nurse you have little say, but you can still ask questions and advocate for the patient. Learn to 'let it go' when someone criticizes you unjustly, and learn from your mistakes when you make them. Observe how things are done and the dynamics of relationships—you will see positive and negative role models. Thank those who help you. Express appreciation for the time they invest in you.*"

—Mishawaka, Indiana; Nursing Instructor

"*Don't be lazy. Stay actively engaged with your patient, your instructor, and the primary nurse.*"

—Pueblo, Colorado; Nursing Instructor

" Most of the health-care team is more than happy to help you learn. Just stay on your toes, do whatever is asked, and ask questions. The health-care team wants to know you are there because you want to be, not because you have to be. "

—**Hughesville, Maryland;** Nursing Student

" Expect the need to prove yourself. Some of the health-care professionals may seem a little standoffish at first. They tend to help the students who show willingness to perform. On the other hand, they seem to ignore those who seem as if they have better things to do than be in clinicals. "

—**Robstown, Texas;** Nursing Student

BE A TEAM PLAYER AND YOU WILL BE REWARDED

As a new student you may feel that you do not have a great deal to offer to the rest of the health-care team. Don't underestimate your fresh pair of eyes and your perception. You may be the person who a patient chooses to open up to about a fear or concern. One of your assessments or observations could be critical to helping treat a patient's illness. Students generally have the time and the benefit of making fresh observations and using their critical thinking skills. If you make an effort to support the work of the nurses and others in the clinical area, you will win their admiration and they will go out of their way to support your learning.

"*Don't get the reputation for sitting at the desk; rather, be out on the unit working with patients or assisting others.*"

—Kansas City, Missouri; Nursing Instructor

"Pick your battles. Sometimes it's better to laugh at yourself and not be perceived as a know-it-all so that you become part of the team. The most important thing for you is to recognize the roles and needs of the people you work with. When everyone works together, patient care benefits. Help others so if you need help the team responds. Be polite, be professional, and take responsibility for all your actions—good and bad."

—**Union Beach, New Jersey;** Nursing Instructor

"Respect the experience of others, but recognize you too have a contribution to make from the very beginning—a new perspective, energy, enthusiasm, and up-to-date knowledge."

—**Fort Worth, Texas;** Nursing Instructor

"*Know what everyone's role is as part of the team. Know how to delegate a task and give positive feedback. Confront in a calm and positive way those who are not carrying their weight, understanding that sometimes we pick up the slack for those who are having a hard time . . . but not all the time.*

Understand that you need to communicate clearly what you expect and what you delegate. Ask the person to repeat what you delegated or expected. My experience has been that most conflicts are due to poor communication.

Don't ask someone to do what you will not do yourself. Get out there and empty bedpans and turn patients when you can. That way on days when you are swamped with paperwork, others will understand that you are not lazy or uncaring, just busy.

Be fair. You can't always make people happy, but if you are fair that is hard to argue with."

—Louisville, Kentucky; Nursing Instructor

"*Realize nurses and doctors are probably working with more patients and fewer staff than they need in order to provide the quality care they would like to provide to their patients. Show them your strengths and how you can help, as well as communicating your learning needs. Don't cluster or mill around in the clinical area. When you are 'caught up' with your patient care, don't sit at the desk or crack open your books. Instead, ask if there is something you can do to help them or some of the other patients (feeding, ambulating, procedures, etc.). Don't criticize what you might see. Know the chain of command. Identify clinical role models and find opportunities to work closely with them.*"

—Fort Gibson, Oklahoma; Nursing Instructor

"*As a student, assume a humble posture. Remember that you are a guest and should act accordingly. However, never be afraid to assert yourself and jump in to help get the work done. Make allies by helping with the nonpatient care activities, and you'll be rewarded by a more robust experience.*"

—Iowa City, Iowa; Nursing Instructor

"*Expect people of all races, origins, accents, and perceptions; and try your best to get along and work with them all, while not forming biased opinions.*"

—Loma Linda, California; Nursing Student

"*We can all push a broom, clean equipment or answer the telephone. Common sense goes a long way. If you have a problem, instead of just complaining, express a solution as well.*"

—Charleston, South Carolina; Nursing Instructor

"*Make sure you know what you want to say prior to speaking. Have the data with you. Demonstrate what you know. Don't let the team intimidate you.*"

—St. Joseph, Missouri; Nursing Instructor

"*Don't let the nurse go too fast!! If you don't understand them, tell them.*"

—Tracy, California; Nursing Instructor

"*Some preceptors will be more than happy to proactively take you by the hand and show and explain everything. Others couldn't care less about you. If the situation is not working to improve your knowledge and skills, ask your clinical instructor to find a new preceptor for you. In the end, what counts is what you learned and can do with confidence, not what a poor preceptor refused to share with you.*"

—West Hartford, Connecticut; Nursing Student

"*Remember it isn't about making friends but about being a good nurse for your patient.*"

—Frankfort, Illinois; Nursing Student

"*Be a patient advocate—always remember that no matter what is going on in the nurse's station or on the unit, the patient should come first. If you keep that in mind, interactions with dietary and physical therapists, etc. will be easier. Be assertive but not aggressive: 'I need you to . . . ' or 'I would appreciate it if . . . . ' I always tell students the nursing assistant can be your best friend or your worst enemy—you decide how you will interact and treat each other. The bed/bath you give today or the help you give will come back later when all heck is breaking out.* **"**

—**Old Bridge, New Jersey;** Nursing Instructor

As a student and as an experienced nurse, you will be working collaboratively with other providers. Some of these team members include physicians, lab techs, patient transporters, nutritionists, and therapists. Each of these individuals will look to you to contribute to patient care and to support the work that they do. While you are in your student experience, make it a point to learn as much as you can about the roles of your colleagues on the team. Find out what each member does to support patient care. Show the members of the team that you are ready, willing, and able to help and to give your best to support their effort. Remember what TEAM stands for: Together Everyone Achieves More. In this care, all efforts should be directed at supporting the patient.

CHAPTER 6

Getting and Giving Report

DOCUMENTATION DOS AND DON'TS THAT LEAD TO CLEAR COMMUNICATION

> " *Nurses need to define what they would want to know about a patient, then deliver that information clearly and concisely, without prejudice.* "
>
> **—Peoria, Illinois;** Nursing Instructor

Almost as important as taking care of your patient is your responsibility to communicate both verbally and in writing about the patient, the care you provided, and the patient's response to care and treatment. In most clinical settings, nurses provide the incoming shift of staff nurses with a verbal report—generally a simple and straightforward account of the patient's status and any exceptional events or concerns that occurred on the prior shift. In some settings, this is done as a group with the entire outgoing shift reporting to the oncoming shift. In other settings, this report may be conducted on a nurse-to-nurse basis while making rounds to the patient's bedside.

In addition to the verbal report, you will be documenting the care you provided in the patient's chart. In both your verbal and written notes, be concise, descriptive, factual, and complete. It is likely your instructor or the clinical unit will have a template or charting system for you to follow. A fairly standard format is the SOAP note. The S stands for *Subjective information*, which may include a direct quote from the patient about how he is feeling or a concern he expressed. The O represents all of the *Objective data* that you collected. It may include the patient's vital signs, fluid intake and output, skin condition, or other observable data. The A stands for your *Assessment* of the patient's status based on the clinical facts. Finally, the P represents the *Plan* for care based on the information you collected. A plan may include contacting a physician, providing pain medication, or any other intervention that will be performed. You may want to review your documentation with your clinical instructor or your staff preceptor until you are comfortable with the process.

"*Getting report: Listen and write down important information. Don't be afraid to ask for information that you need but weren't given (vital signs, lab values, etc.). Don't be embarrassed to ask for clarification if you are unfamiliar with what the RN is telling you. Giving report: Be organized. Use a template to keep your thoughts organized. Practice makes perfect.*"

—Mount Laurel, New Jersey; Nursing Instructor

"*Be brief and specific to what is important information that the next nurse should know about the patient—you don't need to share the entire chart.*"

—Fresno, California; Nursing Student

"*Give clear, organized info. Focus on facts, not judgments.*"

—Sandwich, Massachusetts; Nursing Instructor

"The best advice I received was to document as if you were sitting on a witness stand. Cover all your bases."

—McHenry, Illinois; Nursing Student

"Be prepared and organized. There are many tools out there. For giving report: know the diagnosis, recent vitals, level of pain, significant lab values, impending testing, and the patient's progression through the hospital stay up to this point. Make sure you actually look at the patient before report. (I once took report on a patient who was dead and the nurse didn't know it!) For getting report: have pen and paper in hand, and make sure that all of the above information is given. I like to look at the patient with the off-going nurse before she goes home—that way any loose ends can be fixed before she hits the door."

—Pueblo, Colorado; Nursing Instructor

"Use a recorder, and space out your notes if they are printed so you can add on."

—Kannapolis, North Carolina; Nursing Student

"*Use the SBAR method. S is Situation: what do you need me to know? B is Background: patient history. A is Action: what do you want from the person you call? R is Result: orders, or result of what you need. This can be used for nurse to nurse, or nurse to MD, or nurse to manager.*"

—Dallas, Texas; Nursing Instructor

"*Your documentation should give a clear picture to anyone reading your notes. The man on the moon should be able to understand the picture of the patient after reading your notes.*"

—Pittsburgh, Pennsylvania; Nursing Student

"*Arrive early. Obtain the tools you will need to listen and record your notes in an efficient and orderly manner. Obtain your patient assignment. Quickly scan the physician's orders of each of your patients for the past 24 hours. Walk to the bedside with the off-going nurse and receive report in the patient's room. Involve the patient in the report process. Record your notes. Make quick observations of patient status, equipment, pain level, etc. Ask any questions about patient condition that will be relevant to providing quality care in the next shift—assess wounds, surgical sites, IV sites, etc. Let your patient know you will be returning shortly to perform your assessment and begin care. Ask if he will need you to bring him anything (e.g., pain medication) when you return. Do this for each of your patients.*

After report, you will have a clear idea of how to begin your shift prioritization process. When giving report, collect all meaningful data in advance (intake/output, pain experience, new medications, activity, new orders, etc.). Take the oncoming nurse to the bedside. Give a summary of care for the previous shift, involving the patient in the report process. Allow the nurse time to quickly survey the patient and ask any questions. After report, review orders or pertinent records together."

—Fort Gibson, Oklahoma; Nursing Instructor

"*Keep it relevant; no gossip.*"

—Long Beach, California; Nursing Student

"*Take notes, listen, and ask for missing information. Review report with your clinical instructor to clarify new terminology or unfamiliar procedures prior to starting care. When giving report, check with the clinical facility to see what format is used, and gather all information in an organized, professional manner. Utilize nursing terminology during report. Practice giving report to fellow students; this will help you and them!*"

  —Madison, Indiana; Nursing Instructor

"*Take part in and listen to how nurses give report.*"

  —Vancouver, Washington; Nursing Student

"*When getting report, listen carefully to what the nurse is saying. If something isn't clear, ask the nurse to clarify. The worst thing you can do is walk out of report totally confused.*

When giving report, have a systematic approach. Start with basic patient information, and then focus on the clinical problems/nursing care plans. Be open to questions, and if you don't know something, be honest about it."

  —La Plata, Maryland; Nursing Instructor

"*Only cross out documented mistakes with one line.*"

—**Baltimore, Maryland;** Nursing Student

"*Have everything organized and ready. Give the most important information—please don't give a complete history; they can read the chart. Try not to leave things undone unless you have had a terrible day . . . and then try to stay after to help or apologize for leaving them the mess. And do not make it the norm. Oral report is the best and walking oral is even better—then you can look together.*"

—**Louisville, Kentucky;** Nursing Instructor

"*Use a systems approach, and remember that this is new to you so it's okay if you mess up. Just try to remember the basics.*"

—**Carson, California;** Nursing Student

" Use a 'cheat sheet' to jot down pertinent information from report, then continue to update it during the day as information about the patients is collected. Review in your mind the information about the patients just prior to giving report so the report is clear and concise."

—**Kansas City, Missouri;** Nursing Instructor

" If you do not document it, you did not do it. Document everything as soon as possible because the longer you wait, the more you forget."

—**Baltimore, Maryland;** Nursing Student

" Use a head-to-toe format; be thorough and concise. Verify any info that is not clear to you. If you have computerized documentation, get there 15 minutes early and gather the info yourself so that during the time you are receiving report, you can focus on the info itself, and not on writing fast."

—**Lexington, Kentucky;** Nursing Instructor

"*Learn the format and practice it until it comes naturally without you having to think about it.*"

—St. Michael, Minnesota; Nursing Student

"*Know what you are talking about—organize your data and correlate it. Develop a format for giving the basic information so you can concentrate on giving the updates and changes. Follow through on any orders, diagnostics, change in symptoms, etc. Don't give a problem to the next shift that you haven't at least begun to solve.*

When you get report, make sure you understand what is being conveyed to you; if you don't, ASK QUESTIONS. Appear open and interested in all the information given to you, and avoid being judgmental or opinionated because it shuts down communication. If there is a question, consider walking rounds—you can see firsthand what is going on with the patient."

—Union Beach, New Jersey; Nursing Instructor

"Be precise and accurate. Be honest. Chart everything you did, and don't chart what you didn't do. Little things sometimes affect a lot of things so don't take them for granted."

—**Mesa, Arizona;** Nursing Student

"Establish a plan or format for organizing your information, based on what your facility does. Listen and take notes on what is said. Ask questions for clarification. Keep to the important categories, and don't add in gossip or extraneous material that is not pertinent. Speak positively and confidently. Be clear about what you have done and not done."

—**Mishawaka, Indiana;** Nursing Instructor

"It is good to remember that nursing is a 24-hour job—you might not get to everything, but you must report everything that was done and everything that needs to be done."

—**Sierra Vista, Arizona;** Nursing Student

"*Ask the nurses to slow down and avoid jargon so you can understand the information you are receiving. If there is a written or recorded report, reread or relisten after all the nurses have listened to the report. Use an outline of key information when receiving and giving report.*"

—**Fort Worth, Texas;** Nursing Instructor

"*Be thorough. Start at the head and work your way down. Cover all body systems. Don't forget lab values. Ask important questions: Why is this patient here? What are we doing for her? What is the plan for her? What does she need?*"

—**Wilmington, Delaware;** Nursing Student

"*When receiving report, it is important that the nurse has a clear understanding of the patient's priorities and plan of care. The same is important when giving report—continuing the 'story' of the patient and being able to correlate pathophysiology to clinical manifestations and treatments.*"

—**Baltimore, Maryland;** Nursing Instructor

"*Pick your nurse's brain. Learn shortcuts. Learn what is relevant and keep it short and simple! You won't be perfect right off the bat, but that comes with time.*"

—Orange Park, Florida; Nursing Student

"*Practice, practice, practice. Have nurses and/ or instructors go over them until you are comfortable.*"

—Hughesville, Maryland; Nursing Student

- *Always be organized when giving report.*
- *Give a BRIEF medical background on the client.*
- *Always have forms to take report on; don't rely solely on your memory.*
- *If the student uses the same format for giving report and receiving report, she will be efficient and organized (as well as brief).*

—Mechanicsville, Maryland; Nursing Instructor

> " *Pretend you're writing a story to be read three months from the day the notes are written.* "
>
> **—Mesa, Arizona;** Nursing Student

Learning to effectively document in the patient's record will be a skill that you develop and refine over time. If someone sits down and reads an entire patient record, it should in theory read like a book. The initial assessment and health history should identify the course of the patient's illness and treatment. The progress notes should fill in the details of what happened and how the patient responded to care throughout the hospital stay. The laboratory data and test results supplement the progress notes by tracking the physiological status of the patient. The medication record reflects each and every dose of medication taken by the patient. Chronologically, the chart should give you a mental picture of what happened at each step of the way during the hospital stay.

In your initial days as a student, think about what information *you* would want to know about the patient if you were coming in to provide his care. Take the time to review some progress notes for patients on your unit to get an idea of how to format your documentation. Make sure your handwriting is neat enough to be legible to others. Never make erasures or mark through your writing in a clinical record. The chart is a legal document, so you need to find out how to handle errors in your notes at the particular facility where you are working. And finally, always make sure that you sign and date and record the time of any notation that you make in the patient's record.

CHAPTER 7

Common Mistakes and How to Avoid Them

STUDENTS AND INSTRUCTORS SHARE REAL-LIFE STORIES

"Making a mistake and letting someone know is better than ignoring what happened and taking the worries home with you."

—Baltimore, Maryland; Nursing Student

Despite your best efforts at avoiding them, you will make mistakes as a nurse. Some will be minor and hold limited to no risk for your patients. Other mistakes are serious and warrant detailed follow-up action and improvement of whatever process may have enabled or even supported a mistake. Over the past few years, health-care efforts have focused on recognizing and revamping patient care systems and processes that are error prone. Using good common sense, paying attention to what you are doing, and double-checking on critical procedures will all help you avoid making mistakes. In the event that you knowingly make a mistake anyway, you are obligated to let someone know and to get assistance in determining the impact, if any, on your patient.

MISTAKES I'VE MADE: A STUDENT PERSPECTIVE

In the following examples, fellow students can give you some perspective on errors made in the clinical setting. These examples give you some food for thought about avoiding errors in your own practice. In many of the situations, notice the students advise that paying close attention and focusing on the task at hand may have prevented the errors.

"*In my pediatric rotation I was caring for a child who had a G-tube. I had gotten his feeding ready and was about to hang it when the nurse said, 'What formula is that you're using?' I told her what it was, and she then told me that it was the right brand of formula, but a different calorie content. I felt terrible even though I had not yet hung the feeding, and even if I had it wouldn't have caused harm to him. I learned that even if something looks identical, such as two cans of formula, check and double-check everything."*

—San Antonio, Texas; Nursing Student

"I left the food and drinks of one client next to a confused client who had dysphagia. Before I knew it, the client had eaten a good portion of the food and started to aspirate it. My lesson learned was not only to know your client's medical condition, but also to know the roommate's condition just in case."

—Bayville, New Jersey; Nursing Student

"When hanging a piggyback IV, I didn't put the main saline line under the piggyback, so it never infused in the patient. I recommend slowing down—observe what you have done before you walk away."

—St. Louis, Missouri; Nursing Student

"*Don't be afraid to ask for help with dosage calculations! I was and I almost gave triple the dose. Thankfully my instructor caught my mistake. From then on I always asked to be double-checked, especially when it comes to high-alert medications!*"

—Albuquerque, New Mexico; Nursing Student

"*I documented on the wrong client. Be sure to look at the label before you write. And always look at the patient's armband and ask the name before you do anything. This is very important. I almost removed an IV from the wrong patient.*"

—Floresville, Texas; Nursing Student

"*There was a miscommunication between me and the primary nurse, and two incompatible medications were mixed in an IV, and a precipitate formed. I learned about taking time to give a clear report when going on breaks, and I learned what a precipitate really looks like and what to do about it.*"

—Madison, Wisconsin; Nursing Student

"*I did not check pedal pulses on a patient because I did not know how during a head-to-toe assessment. For the next patient, I got the nerve to ask someone. She showed me and told me to practice. I felt bad that I did not check the prior patient's pulses. I also felt bad that I did not have the courage to ask from the beginning. NEVER be afraid to ask questions. It benefits everyone. I will never forget when my preceptor told me, 'I would be more scared of a nurse who thinks she knows everything than a nurse who doesn't and asks questions.'*"

—North Aurora, Illinois; Nursing Student

"*With my instructor in front of me, I could not remember that I needed gloves before doing a finger stick test. She finally told me what I was missing. I always remembered after that to put on my gloves.*"

—Santa Clara, California; Nursing Student

"*I had two patients in side-by-side rooms. I had the medication for one of them, and I was rushing and entered the wrong room. Thankfully, even before checking the bracelet of my patient, I realized that I was in the wrong room. Pay attention and be focused!*"

—**South Yarmouth, Massachusetts;** Nursing Student

"*I forgot to give a patient his Coumadin because of the placement of the order on the MAR (medication record). I was working nights for this particular clinical rotation, and the sheet was divided into days and nights by a dotted line. For some reason, my 1900 med was placed on the day side, and I did not check that side of the sheet and received a med error. My patient received the Coumadin, however it was given a few hours later. Check your entire MAR!*"

—**Lancaster, California;** Nursing Student

"*I was trying to squeeze air out of a saline syringe to flush an IV and it slipped and I squirted the patient. From now on, I squeeze the air out away from the patient!*"

—**Rockville, Maryland;** Nursing Student

"*I didn't flush an IV site before going to get blood to hang. Always flush an IV site at the beginning of the shift if you don't have an infusion going.*"

—**Arrowsmith, Illinois;** Nursing Student

"*I almost administered the incorrect dose of a med. I had double-checked the MAR to the meds and I discovered it. I was honest about it to my nurse and my instructor. Be honest! It's the ONLY way to go. If you're not, people will not trust you, and it can bring your dreams of becoming or being a nurse to a halt.*"

—**Fremont, California;** Nursing Student

"*I forgot to sign the MAR after giving a medication. In nursing, if it is not documented, it was not done. Always document.*"

—**Allentown, Pennsylvania;** Nursing Student

"*I had a needle stick injury in my last clinical rotation in nursing school. I was sitting next to the patient, going through her many meds (she was elderly) while she was sitting in a chair, and I administered a heparin injection while sitting down. I swabbed with alcohol, pinched her abdomen, and poked with the needle, which went right through her skin fold and into my finger on the other side. Make sure to always wear gloves, and stand while doing this to administer more straight on. If you do stick yourself, IRRIGATE IMMEDIATELY then report to employee health right away. Fortunately, the patient was negative of all organisms and so was I.*"

—**Alexandria, Virginia;** Nursing Student

"*In my first clinical, I was so anxious when my instructor was in the vicinity that I would often tremble uncontrollably. One time, I drew up 20 units of regular insulin rather than 2 units. I was devastated when I found out what I had done. I will never forget that mistake, and I will never make it again. As students, we will make mistakes, but these mistakes will help us learn and grow as nurses.*"

—**Pasadena, California;** Nursing Student

"*I put up the bed rails clear around the patient instead of only the top two rails. The nurse quietly lowered the two rails by the foot of the bed, and we discussed this outside of the patient room. Praise in public and correct in private.*"

—**Lenoir City, Tennessee;** Nursing Student

"*The very first time I did a straight catheter, I broke sterile field and had to repeat the procedure. I was very nervous, but my professor and the nurse I was working with were great and allowed me to do it again and complete it correctly.*"

—**Baltimore, Maryland;** Nursing Student

"*I made an inappropriate joke in front of one of the nurses who was offended by it. I learned to grow up and take nursing more seriously.*"

—**Shepherdstown, West Virginia;** Nursing Student

"*I was talking to a patient about his condition and it was the wrong patient. Before I start my day, I clarify which is bed 1 and which is bed 2 when patients share a room.*"

—Newburg, Maryland; Nursing Student

"*I was caring for two female newborns. I gave the correct injection to baby A, yet I documented the injection in baby B's chart. Both newborns had the same first name. I learned to pay special attention to chart names.*"

—Burleson, Texas; Nursing Student

"*A patient in the ICU had multiple IVs. The IV started beeping, and I turned off the wrong IV pump. I didn't catch it until an hour later! Thank goodness it didn't harm the patient, but it has made me more vigilant about IVs.*"

—Rohnert Park, Texas; Nursing Student

"I was emptying a Foley catheter in the middle of a clinical day. I measured the urine and left the room to document the output. When I entered the room several minutes later, I realized that I had not closed the valve on the reservoir. I learned to always check to make sure the valve is closed. It is not a good idea to rush—I ended up spending, not saving, time. I had a mess to clean up which took some time. I also had to change the Foley because the closed system had been left opened, which put the patient at risk for infection."

—**Robstown, Texas;** Nursing Student

"I stuck myself with a sterile needle when I was drawing up meds for a patient. I was so nervous, plus I had little experience with syringes. The five-minute lab at school does not prepare you for the real world. After that, I came home and practiced removing caps off needles over and over again."

—**Social Circle, Georgia;** Nursing Student

"*When I made the mistakes that stand out in my mind, I knew instantly that they were caused by rushing and being more concerned about finishing than doing something carefully. Most of all, I realized that I needed to be honest and report incidents, even if nobody knew what had happened at the time. Yes, I was embarrassed that I had forgotten my instructions. But patient safety is the priority, and your coworkers need to know that they can trust you to be honest.*"

—**Philadelphia, Pennsylvania;** Nursing Student

"*During my senior practicum, I actually made two mistakes that were thankfully non–life threatening. The first mistake: I hung a patient's IV med but forgot to open the IV line to the patient. Therefore, the patient did not get the med until I went in about an hour later (when the med was supposed to be done infusing) and realized that it had not run. From this, I learned that it is important to assess prior to leaving.*

The second mistake: I hung a med above the level of the NS when it was supposed to be the other way around, again causing the med not to infuse. From this, I learned that it is important to look up the med and nursing considerations prior to entering a patient's room so that you're going by fact and not recall!"

—**Baltimore, Maryland;** Nursing Student

"After drawing blood from a patient, I used the stickers from the patient's file to label the tubes and send them to the lab. Unfortunately, the stickers in my patient's file belonged to another patient. I learned that I need to recheck everything."

—**Olathe, Kansas;** Nursing Student

"I had the opportunity to watch my patient have a cardiac cath. When the physician started quizzing me about cardiac things, I had no clue as to the answers. I also didn't know what to do to care for the patient. I learned to read up on procedures that are common on the floor that I was assigned to."

—**La Porte, Texas;** Nursing Student

SOME COMMON MISTAKES I'VE SEEN: AN INSTRUCTOR PERSPECTIVE

In the following comments, clinical instructors discuss their views on errors that they have witnessed among their students. One of the most common suggestions you'll notice reinforces the need for you to be prepared in advance for clinical. Another is to pay close and careful attention to details and to following the proper steps in completing procedures such as medication administration. Try to develop good habits and safe habits at the beginning of your experience.

"*Some mistakes I've witnessed:*

● *Lack of personal responsibility—the whole 'you didn't tell me I had to do exactly that' issue. Students need to understand that when a faculty person tells them to be familiar with the teaching needs of a patient population, they mean all of the teaching outlined in the text, not just the first one on a list. Personal responsibility is critical for nurses: if it isn't your personal professional responsibility as a nurse, who do you think is going to take care of that aspect of patient care? Faculty don't expect students to be experts, but we do expect thorough preparation.*

- *Lack of follow-through on what they learned in previous semesters or courses, and knowledge that those learnings are applicable in other clinical situations. Consider that everything you learn you will use again and again in each subsequent course, clinical experience, and semester.*

- *Blowing off details as unimportant. Nursing is about the details. If you are supposed to do a head-to-toe assessment on a patient, but she is busy with visitors, you are still responsible for doing the head-to-toe. Being nice is fine, and having a happy patient is good, but a happy patient that is bleeding to death is not good.*

- *Making assumptions. Assumptions such as all patients are straight (heterosexual), or all patients read English, or all patients understand what you mean when you do teaching are insulting at best and dangerous at times. Begin by asking respectful questions to assess your starting point, then go into whatever else you have to do (family assessment, patient education, discharge teaching, etc.)."*

—St. Paul, Minnesota; Nursing Instructor

"*Students often have an incorrect knowledge of medications—dose, action, etc. They should carry a drug book with them if possible and look up medications beforehand to be prepared. Poor documentation is also a problem. Students should review their thoughts and write on scrap paper before putting them in the chart, especially if it's a long, completed note. They should also carry a pocket dictionary if spelling is a problem.*"

—**Philadelphia, Pennsylvania;** Nursing Instructor

"*There are always medication errors. Take your time. Follow the five rights: right patient, right time, right drug, right dose, right route. Poor time management makes for late entries in charting, and possibly late-given medications. Pace yourself and plan out your activities. Prioritize. Students have difficulty making choices of who/what to do first. This comes with experience. The more practice they can get the better.*"

—**Bakersfield, California;** Nursing Instructor

"*I see many student nurses rely on technology and not on their skills and common sense. I always remind my students to 'treat the patient, not the monitor.' I often relay to them a story where a patient was nearly defibrillated because the monitor showed asystole, when in fact a lead had come off. The patient was awake, alert, oriented, pink, warm, and dry. These symptoms are not generally associated with asystole. I think that student nurses are afraid they will make a mistake if they trust their skills. My advice is to not only try to learn the skills presented during school, but remember your common sense. If the patient does not seem to be in distress, he probably is not; just as if the patient seems in distress, it does not matter what the monitor may say—help your patient.*"

—Lubbock, Texas; Nursing Instructor

"*I come across many communication errors between the nurse taking care of the patient and the student. Students are afraid to ask questions, hesitate, and then later find out they did not have all the details about the patient situation, but were too afraid to ask. My advice would be: don't be afraid to ask questions. You need to ask questions to learn. By not asking questions, you are really decreasing your ability to learn through the situation.*"

—Rock Hill, South Carolina; Nursing Instructor

"*One error I encounter is that students don't follow the proper steps for medication administration. They don't verify the patient with two identifiers before giving medication. I would encourage new nursing students to practice the process of checking the armband before giving the medications.*"

—Atlanta, Georgia; Nursing Instructor

"*Most common errors:*

1. Medication knowledge prior to administration of the drug. Errors include lack of assessment regarding pertinent laboratory values and diagnostic test results that may affect administration of the medication, and lack of research about potential interactions of various medications.

2. *Medication knowledge during administration of the drug. Students always need to continue to do the basic 'five rights' of medication administration, because at times they are not sure about actual administration of the medication (i.e., length of time of administration, potential adverse reactions that may occur during or immediately after administration of the drug).*

3. *Failure to review the patient's medical records to update medication information (health-care provider orders, pertinent lab results). A medication is sometimes given when it has been discontinued or when it is contraindicated.*

4. *Failure to follow the standards of care of the institution when caring for clients. Even though the textbooks may have general guidelines, it is critical to follow the SOCs for the institution where the student is practicing.*

5. *Lack of communication with the primary nurse and other health-care providers in the acute care setting. Sometimes there is confusion about roles and responsibilities, and this can be dangerous, especially when it deals with medication administration. Other problems that I have seen*

*due to this include lack of ambulation, post-op
activities, and daily-living activities that increase
client comfort.*

My advice:

*1, 2, and 3: Review all medications thoroughly before
clinical, especially monitoring. That is necessary. If
a client is receiving a potassium wasting diuretic
or a corticosteroid, it makes sense to monitor the
serum potassium! Use the basic five rights and
check them three times with EVERY medication.
Research has shown that most medication errors
are due to failure to do this. Check the health-care
provider orders frequently—definitely before the
administration of medications.*

*4 and 5: Obtain a copy of standard orders prior to
clinical. Ask the staff questions about standards
of care prior to clinical. Make up a 'game plan'
with the primary nurse in the morning, so the
plan of care and division of duties are clear. Clarify
what needs to be reported to the primary nurse
(e.g., appearance of surgical incision, tolerance of
ambulation, etc.).*"

—De Pere, Wisconsin; Nursing Instructor

"*Med errors affect both students and RNs most commonly. To avoid med errors it is imperative for students to develop the habit of triple-checking meds: at the time of removal, at the med room, and at the bedside. Another common mistake I see is not completing assignments on time. Without completing the assignments the student cannot be prepared to learn the curriculum.*"

—**Escondido, California;** Nursing Instructor

"*Students often have the inability to differentiate between two different patient scenarios, although they may have similar interventions. This is, in essence, critical thinking. My best advice I give to students is to have them ask 'why' I am doing something as opposed to 'what' I should do in a given situation.*"

—**Salt Lake City, Utah;** Nursing Instructor

"*My advice is to learn as much as you can about medications before administering them. Check and double-check. I often see errors in charting. Learn proper charting for the facility you are working at. Don't be too proud to ask questions.*"

—**Centennial, Colorado;** Nursing Instructor

- *Late or incomplete interventions due to poor time management. When students only have one patient to take care of, they try to stretch things out so they don't get bored. When they are challenged to take more than one patient, that comes back to haunt them because they don't know how to coordinate care between patients and they don't know how to do things efficiently. I push my third-semester students to work on efficiency first and then we begin to add patients to the assignment by mid-semester.*

- *Incomplete or inaccurate assessments. I find that few students come out of their basic assessment course with the ability to perform an organized head-to-toe assessment and accurately document their findings. I spend a lot of time reteaching these skills. I like to start the semester with a skills lab where we go over each portion of a basic assessment, identifying norms and abnormal findings and how to document each. We then practice on one another until the assessment can be completed and documented in 15 minutes or less. In clinical, I follow this up by not allowing A.M. meds to be given until the student does an initial assessment on the patient and documents it to my satisfaction. This has really helped to curtail the tendency of students to assess one or two things each time they go in the room (as they think of them), rather than doing it all at once.*

—Dallas, Texas; Nursing Instructor

"*Nerves, feelings of insecurity, and—most seriously—being poorly prepared prevent students from thinking critically and lead to significant errors and omissions. Prepare and study carefully! Recognize that caring for another human is both the ultimate privilege AND responsibility.*"

—Rochester, Minnesota; Nursing Instructor

The issue of making mistakes in clinical practice is a tricky one to consider and discuss with you as a novice. On the one hand, you do not want to become paralyzed with fear or so paranoid that you are afraid to take action. On the other hand, there is a reality that some errors can be serious or even fatal for patients. That is why it is imperative that you think before you act. Consider the patient's safety and well-being at all times. If something does not seem right about your equipment, the patient's condition, or the action you are about to take, then stop, think, and check into the situation. Common nursing routines, such as administering medications, have numerous steps built in to ensure that errors are minimized or avoided. However, none of these steps will secure the well-being of your patient if you do not follow through with them. Be prepared and be alert, and you will have set the stage for effective and safe practice.

CHAPTER 8

How to Deal with Your Stress

HOW TO LET YOURSELF TAKE A DEEP BREATH AND RELAX

"*Learn to laugh at yourself (and your instructors—although not in front of them, please)!*"

—Philadelphia, Pennsylvania; Nursing Instructor

"*Remember that you will have some good weeks and some bad weeks.*"

—Norfolk, Nebraska; Nursing Student

If you are feeling stressed, you are in the right place. School is stressful, and a nursing major always cranks that stress up a few notches. While your friends and roommates are sleeping in or skipping class, you are up at the crack of dawn, wearing your uniform and going to clinical somewhere. While everyone else can party or put that paper off until the last minute, you have to be prepared. To some degree, stress helps our minds and our bodies prepare and remain on the edge of readiness—remember the old "fight or flight" response? However, too much stress and you can do yourself in . . . and maybe even fall to pieces. The trick is to find a balance so you can manage your stress as you cope with the situation of being a new player in the health-care world. Take the time out to balance your life, your home, your family, your job (if you have one), and your studies. The time you spend will be well worth it.

REMEMBER WHY YOU'RE THERE

Nursing is a wonderful job. You will have a broad set of job opportunities, the promise of available positions, and lots of flexibility in terms of work settings and work hours. You can do well *and* do good at the same time. You do need to work at making it to the finish line, which hopefully involves getting good grades and of course, passing the NCLEX exam to earn your RN license. The license will be your finish line, so use the time in your classes and clinical to prepare yourself to get there.

"*Remember that you have chosen the very best profession in the world. There are not many jobs where you can look in the mirror at the end of a work day and see a person who has made someone's life better—every single day. Find that excitement and joy. Love what you are doing! Share what you are doing with others. Find a classmate, friend, or family member who you can vent to when things get difficult. Talk to a professor who is totally joyful and upbeat about nursing, and ask how he or she got through the difficult times. (They did have some, you know!)*"

—Pueblo, Colorado; Nursing Instructor

"*I kept my eyes on the goal of becoming a nurse.*"

—Riverside, New Jersey; Nursing Student

"*I said to myself: This is a journey that I initiated and that I want to participate in. This is not punishment.*"

—San Jose, California; Nursing Student

EDIT YOUR PERSONAL LIFE AS THOROUGHLY AS POSSIBLE

Temporary sacrifices have probably been very real for you by now. You are spending money, time, and energy on nursing school. You may need to reevaluate your priorities once again as you move into clinical experiences. Hopefully you can call together some additional support to assist you with this critical time in your program. Try to find out about all of the available funding for your program. Scholarships and student loans may help cover living expenses so that you can cut back on your work hours. Look ahead to your entire program and figure out what you need to do to make school your number one priority until you get that degree or diploma.

"Do not expect to work full-time and be a successful nursing student. Take out loans if you need to, but don't try to work more than 20 hours a week (and many students can't work that much). Make sure your family members all understand the time commitment of nursing education. Enlist friends who have completed the program who come from a similar cultural background to explain the time *required to your family. Expect to have a severely diminished social life while in nursing school. Tell friends that you'll call (and then do it every few weeks) and get together over semester or summer break to catch up."*

—St. Paul, Minnesota; Nursing Instructor

"I would not recommend working, if possible. I did both, and the semesters that I worked were unbearable."

—Jacksonville, Florida; Nursing Student

"Realize that nursing school is more time and energy demanding than most other programs of study. Be honest with yourself as to whether this is the best time for you to be in school. If your children are very young, if you are already a caregiver to a frail adult, if you are having significant problems in your marriage or other relationship, if you work long hours at your present job with little likelihood of being able to reduce your hours (or even quit), this may not be the best time to go to nursing school. This is a

conversation I have had with many students over the years. If waiting a year or so would be more likely to ensure your success, wait.

If family members are very supportive (as I hope they are), take them up on their offers to cook meals, clean your house, keep your children, etc., to allow you time to study. Since the majority of nursing students are still women, realize that women have developed an idea over the years that we are supposed to martyr ourselves to everything we do. Be a little more assertive and tell others how they can help, and then thank them for doing so. Use stress-reduction strategies that have worked in the past. But realize that the stressors you will encounter will probably be different from what you have experienced in the past. Realize, too, that as you move through your program, you will develop strategies that will smooth out the path. The first term is always the hardest."

—Southside, Alabama; Nursing Instructor

"*Know going in that nursing school is very difficult and very time-consuming. Prepare your family for your 'absence' so that you don't get caught between school and life (but always remember to make time for yourself!).*"

—La Plata, Maryland; Nursing Instructor

"*Don't work unless you have to. And if you have to, get a job as a patient care tech or CNA if at all possible. This will increase your learning curve. Health-care entities will also be more willing to work with your school schedule.*"

—Dallas, Texas; Nursing Instructor

"*Nursing school needs to be a priority. I often counsel students that it needs to be the right time in their lives to undertake the rigors of school. Many students try to juggle too many roles and I reinforce that nursing school is physically, intellectually, and emotionally draining, and that they need to be in a place where they have the time and energy to tackle it!*"

—Salt Lake City, Utah; Nursing Instructor

BE PREPARED AND PLAN AHEAD

The best thing you can do to support your role as a student nurse is to immerse yourself in your studies. When you start a new clinical course, read through the entire course guide or syllabus. Keep your assignments noted on a calendar. Get going on projects or assignments in advance, and avoid the panic that comes with last-minute work. If you leave things to the very end, you will not give yourself the chance to edit, revise, and polish your material.

"*A good way to combat anxiety about school is to do what you are supposed to do—read the material, complete assignments, come to class, participate in learning exercises, and review study questions from NCLEX review books to practice for unit exams. When you* know *that you have done the work to learn the material, you aren't so anxious that someone might ask you a question about something you have only scanty knowledge about.*"

—Fort Gibson, Oklahoma; Nursing Instructor

"*By becoming an organized person, you can decrease stress significantly. I was not an organized person when I entered nursing school, and I quickly caused much more stress for myself than necessary. I found that by taking just a little time (I used Sunday afternoon) to get prepared for the week ahead, I was much less stressed as the week progressed.*

Another benefit of time management is that it facilitates other activities. Moderation is very important during school and life. You have to continue to do the things that make you happy while in school or you will go insane, but obviously the frequency of fun activities may reduce. By managing your time well, it is much easier to plan for fun events or hobbies. For example, you will know well in advance that if you want to go to a party on Saturday night, you have to work a little harder every day the previous week until then (as opposed to realizing you are behind on Saturday afternoon). Take responsibility for your life and make decisions accordingly."

—Lubbock, Texas; Nursing Instructor

"Front-load your semester, meaning do as much up front as you can so that the last few weeks of the semester you have less to do when you have a tendency to be more stressed."

—Charleston, South Carolina; Nursing Instructor

"Never avoid work—go straight at it and get it done. If you want to avoid work, you should choose another profession."

—Iowa City, Iowa; Nursing Instructor

"Life happens. You must be prepared for the unexpected because it will happen as soon as you begin nursing school."

—Charlotte, North Carolina; Nursing Instructor

"*It's okay to be nervous when you are doing something new. Your instructor understands that completely. What gets you into trouble is when you are nervous because you are unprepared. That makes you dangerous on clinical, and no one wants an unsafe situation. Read, read, read—your book, journals, Internet sites, newsletters, etc. The more you know about nursing and trends, the easier it will be to understand the particulars of what you need to do with your own patients. Negative thinking and worrying saps your energy. Think about and build on the positives you have already accomplished—no matter how small. Each success is a building block for the foundation of your ultimate goal!*"

—Union Beach, New Jersey; Nursing Instructor

"*Dealing with stress during nursing school and clinical was accomplished mainly by keeping on task, completing assignments ahead of time and not waiting until the last minute, keeping a planner of times and due dates, and keeping school and family in perspective.*"

—Peterson, Minnesota; Nursing Student

KNOW THAT YOU HAVE A REASON TO BE STRESSED!

It is important to give yourself permission to be stressed while you are in clinical. Unless you have worked in health care before, just being in the hustle-bustle world of a hospital and around sick people will be a new and different experience. The sights, sounds, and experiences will overstimulate your senses. So take care of yourself and be ready to accept the newness of the situation. Do you know how you generally react to new and stressful situations? Whatever the response is for you, it will likely be your customary pattern. Plan ahead. Do you have ideas and suggestions for yourself about the best and most functional ways that you respond to stress?

"*Recognize that nursing is not cognitively structured like other learning situations, and you will be forced to think and study like you have not done before. Thinking like a nurse requires you to use a part of your thought process that is not typically used in education.*"

—**Durham, North Carolina;** Nursing Instructor

"*I would like to suggest to incoming nursing students to first think of nursing as a scientific profession that requires a commitment that other professions do not command. New students should be allowed to formulate their own impressions about nursing, rather than get advice from senior students' 'horror stories.' These can be precursors to undue stress. Each individual deals with stress differently. In my opinion the best way to reduce stress is to be prepared on an ongoing basis.*"

—**St. Louis, Missouri;** Nursing Instructor

USE ALL SOUNDING BOARDS AVAILABLE

You will find that your fellow students can be a great support group as you move through nursing school. Consider ideas such as a study group or a group that meets for lunch or rides together to clinical. Use this time to support your classmates—teaching content to someone else is a great way to reinforce your own learning. You may want to form a group and invite a faculty member to join you. If you are feeling that your stress level is getting out of control, find out if there is a guidance counselor or student coaching center at your college or university.

"*Talk with someone about how you are feeling—preferably someone who has similar experience, but not on the same unit.*"

—**Baltimore, Maryland;** Nursing Instructor

"*My nursing friends were my lifeline. We studied together, cried together, and socialized together.*"

—**Evergreen Park, Illinois;** Nursing Student

"*Use your peers as sounding boards. I know of many students who have run into family stress because their families don't really understand what they're going through, and who never dreamed it would be as hard as it is. Other nursing students are excellent supports.*"

—**Manalapan, New Jersey;** Nursing Instructor

"*Be patient with yourself. Avail yourself of campus services offered to help with anxiety and stress, and do it early. Do not wait until you get into your last semesters before doing this—each semester gets harder as you go through the curriculum.*"

—Naperville, Illinois; Nursing Instructor

"*Talk to a nurse you know or one in your family. Knowing that others have been in your shoes or just having someone to vent to who has been there helps. They survived and you will too. Make a list of what you want to do with your degree and why you decided to go back to school, and keep it where you will see it every day.*"

—Louisville, Kentucky; Nursing Instructor

"*The most helpful thing was peer support from fellow classmates—lots of it! It's very important to bond with peers, because only someone going through it can truly appreciate the experience— the stress, the anxiety, and the accomplishment— like no other loved one ever could.*"

—Collingswood, New Jersey; Nursing Student

KNOW YOURSELF AND DEVISE METHODS THAT WORK FOR *YOU*

Coping with stress is an individual skill. What stresses one person out may be a piece of cake to another. Likewise, your methods of responding to stress and relieving it are likely to be unique to you and your personality type. Some people like to work out, others like to curl up and rest. It is helpful to know what works for you (not your best friend or your sister) and plan it into your schedule on a regular basis.

"*To deal with the stress of nursing school, I set aside one to two hours a day for reading or homework after my children went to bed. Keeping my study dates would keep me organized which led to less stress. Also, I would reward myself weekly with shopping or eating out with my friends if I kept up with my homework.*"

—Sapulpa, Oklahoma; Nursing Student

"*I took it one day at a time and just made sure I knew what I needed to know . . . and if I didn't know something, I would look it up ASAP so as not to stress myself out about not knowing.*"

—**Tracy, California;** Nursing Student

"*I didn't listen to other students stress out. By ignoring their stresses, I didn't overinflate mine.*"

—**Indianapolis, Indiana;** Nursing Student

"*I relaxed in a hot bath while reviewing the night before a big exam.*"

—**Jacksonville, Florida;** Nursing Student

"*I kept thinking positively and always kept telling myself that I am smart, competent, and confident.*"

—**Allentown, Pennsylvania;** Nursing Student

"*I believe getting a lot of sleep allowed me to stay focused in class, have daily energy, and reduced my chances of getting ill.*"

—**Vernon, Connecticut;** Nursing Student

"*I prayed (a lot) for patience and strength! I had an infant, a toddler, and a teenager at home while going through nursing school. If I can do it anyone can!!*"

—**Kokomo, Indiana;** Nursing Student

EVERYBODY NEEDS SOME TIME AWAY

An important time to build into your routine is some downtime for yourself. Time management gurus generally recommend that you schedule one day or half day a week for a date with yourself. This may prove to be a luxury while you are in school, but even an hour a day or every couple of days will help you regroup.

"I've always been a musical and athletic person. When I had free time or I felt stressed out, I would go for a run, play basketball, listen to some music, or go play the piano. It really relaxes me when I do something that I love."

—Edinburg, Texas; Nursing Student

"Have some fun, if even for 30 minutes, every day."

—St. Joseph, Missouri; Nursing Instructor

"Get selfish. Make time for yourself. Make a date with yourself to do just what you want. Include sleep in your schedule. Make sure friends and family honor your time limits. Excuse yourself from attending events that will cause you to miss study or sleep time. Do not answer the phone unless you have the time to talk. Let the answering devices or voice mail work for you, and let your family and friends know to expect you to NOT RETURN CALLS until you have time."

—Longview, Texas; Nursing Instructor

"*When I felt completely stressed out I just stepped away from the books and treated myself—either to a nice dinner with friends and family, or I went to the gym and walked my stress off! I found that to be a great way to relax.*"

—Cherry Hill, New Jersey; Nursing Student

"*When I had a bad test or bad day of clinical I would allow myself to rest the next day.*"

—Danville, Illinois; Nursing Student

"*I had a four-hour commute every day back and forth from school. I used that time to relieve some stress and relax. I also used some of that time to listen to lectures . . . not too much, though, because after sitting in lecture and running around all day during clinical, the last thing I wanted to do was to take it on the road with me. I used that time as stress relief. Driving was my therapy. My car literally became a place that I called home. I ate breakfast, lunch, and dinner in it, my friends and I studied in it, and I slept in it during break. It was great.*"

—Anaheim, California; Nursing Student

"*To be honest, when studying for tests I did not just read or practice questions in a quiet area. I would watch TV between 15-minute study intervals. It's weird, but it worked for someone who stressed really easy. During the breaks I would watch TV, but really I would think about what I just read or the questions I answered wrong and the rationales.*"

—**San Antonio, Texas;** Nursing Student

"*If I found myself getting too frustrated while at clinical or when doing clinical paperwork, I would remove myself from the situation for a few minutes and mentally prepare myself to continue.*"

—**Defiance, Ohio;** Nursing Student

"*I took one day off a week and would not let myself open books or think about school.*"

—**Palmdale, California;** Nursing Student

> " *I survived by not living, breathing, and eating nursing school. You have to give yourself some away time.* "
>
> **—Atlanta, Georgia;** Nursing Student

In every chapter of this book, the experts have pointed out that nursing is both rewarding and challenging. At the same time, it's a fact that nursing school and clinical experiences are also stressful. You will be doing yourself a favor now by developing some healthy outlets and ways to cope with the stress. You may already know what works for you. If you don't, try some new ideas, such as physical exercise, meditation, fine arts, or even watching a movie or TV. You will have more to give to others if you take good care of yourself first.

CHAPTER 9

How Your Professors Can Guide the Way

UTILIZING THE PROFESSIONAL RESOURCES THAT ARE RIGHT IN FRONT OF YOU

"One of the most important things students can learn from faculty is how to learn."

—**Baltimore, Maryland;** Nursing Instructor

As with people you meet in most areas of life, there will be nursing faculty that you connect with on a personal level and those that you do not connect with. Believe it or not, you can learn a great deal from both groups. Hopefully you can identify a faculty member who you admire, relate to, and can establish a bond with. Faculty nurses enter the education profession because they enjoy helping students learn, and they will take pride in having a new, highly motivated student seek them out as a mentor. Make the most of resource people like this in your educational program. Today's mentor or "go-to person" can easily become tomorrow's reference for a new job or a recommendation for graduate school. In this section, our experienced students and faculty share some ideas on how to get the most out of the student/faculty relationship.

FIND THE PROFESSOR WHO SPEAKS YOUR LANGUAGE

You will be spending a great deal of time with nursing faculty—in lecture, discussion groups, and clinical settings. Faculty members have unique personalities and quirks just like everyone else. It is likely that some faculty will motivate your learning and provide solid support to you as an individual more than others. Take the time to reach out and get to know these key faculty members. Seek them out when you are struggling, even if you are fundamentally questioning your academic decision to become a nurse. Some students consider talking with faculty to be a form of "sucking up" or solicitous behavior. Nothing could be further from the truth. Faculty can become lifelong sources of professional mentoring and advice. If you plan to advance in your area of practice, forming networking relationships with faculty can be a major source of support.

"The most successful students find an instructor who they can communicate well with and develop a relationship that is similar to a mentoring relationship. Communication is key. The student who 'hides' from the instructor is likely to get lower grades, less attention, and less of an education. Ask questions—in class, in the clinical setting, in the hallway, during office hours—any time but 2 A.M. on a cell phone. Prepare for class work and clinical experiences by writing down questions that are relevant to the topic when reviewing books, patient charts, and handouts."

—**Pueblo, Colorado;** Nursing Instructor

"If there is one mentor or professor who you really can relate to or click with, don't hesitate to use his or her knowledge and expertise."

—**Cherry Hill, New Jersey;** Nursing Student

"Faculty/student mentoring is best achieved when students select a faculty member they are comfortable with."

—**Oklahoma City, Oklahoma;** Nursing Instructor

"Pay attention—each professor tends to have her own style. You pick which style is most comfortable for you and build upon it."

—**Baltimore, Maryland;** Nursing Student

"One of my professors was my rock; I could turn to her for anything and everything. You need that. Get to know at least one of your professors and have that professional and personal relationship that will span the years. Talk to them if you are having difficulties; they will listen. Believe it or not, they really do care, at least most of them."

—**Corpus Christi, Texas;** Nursing Student

"More than likely you will find a professor or two who you can really relate to, and that professor may become more of a mentor for you, but I think every professor can in some way be a resource. Do not be afraid to take advantage of them."

—**Mokena, Illinois;** Nursing Student

"*It helped me to call them for venting when needed.*"

—**Louisville, Kentucky;** Nursing Student

PROFESSORS LIKE TO ANSWER QUESTIONS, SO ASK!

The student years are a great time to cultivate the practice of getting support for your information and skill needs. Rather than a sign of weakness, knowing when and how to get information that you need is a talent and a skill in its own right. Faculty are disappointed when students perform poorly or make repeated mistakes with papers, care plans, or projects but never seek input or advice. Most likely your education is a cost to you, both in money and time. You will get the most out of the experience if you seek out help and input in advance.

"*Students need to ask questions of their professors. As we go through the material, students often become lost and do not have a complete understanding of the concepts. Very few ask for clarification. I think students don't understand that teachers love to get questions; it allows clarification for the whole group.*"

—**Charlotte, North Carolina;** Nursing Instructor

"*Ask for feedback after clinicals and papers—how could you have done better?*"

—**Valley Stream, New York;** Nursing Student

"*Don't wait until the last minute to ask for help.*"

—**Louisville, Kentucky;** Nursing Instructor

"*Ask questions. Know the 'hows,' but ask the 'whys.' Not only will they be happy that you are a knowledge seeker, but this also translates into patient safety, and who doesn't love that?*"

—**Stow, Ohio;** Nursing Student

"*Always ask questions. When you stop asking questions is when you become an unsafe nurse/ nursing student.*"

—**Tacoma, Washington;** Nursing Student

PROFESSORS ARE RESOURCES FOR CAREER PLANNING

In the midst of a variety of clinical settings and different types of patients, you may become a bit overwhelmed as you start to think about your own career as a nurse. Do you want pediatrics, med-surg, the OR? The good news is that you will have a broad base of opportunities for specialization or career focus. The other good news is that you can always shift gears and expand your career in a different direction. Your faculty can help you as you consider your future career options. Your clinical instructors can help you consider the ins and outs of specialty practice roles, both in the hospital and in a community setting.

"*Perform a self-analysis of strengths and weaknesses, and clarify these with the faculty to determine the best work situation after graduation.*"

—**Kansas City, Missouri;** Nursing Instructor

"*You need to stay in touch with your professors because you need references, advice, and solace. Don't burn your bridges because you will need to cross them again.*"

—**Pennington, New Jersey;** Nursing Student

"*Many students have questions about career path choices regarding subspecialty areas and continuing education for advanced degrees, in addition to expectations of the real world versus school settings. Instructors/professors should be able to guide or refer students to the appropriate resources or colleagues in different subspecialty areas and should have an idea about local hospital hiring practices, pay scales, and work requirements (rotating shifts, holidays, weekends, etc.).*"

—**Charleston, South Carolina;** Nursing Instructor

"*Find what things they like best about nursing or what is most interesting to them. This is where their knowledge lies.*"

—**Chandler, Arizona;** Nursing Student

PROFESSORS WILL HELP YOU THINK LIKE A NURSE

Nurses need to learn to think critically and apply the scientific method in their work with patients. You use your senses to observe and collect information. You collect more information and sometimes measure physiologic responses. You provide treatment and care based on available data and clinical decision-making. You communicate with other nurses and with patients, and then you evaluate the impact of care and treatment. Applying this process is a multidimensional and multifaceted activity. Remember that it is a new process for you, and you may not be totally aware of what step to take next or how to interpret the information that you have at your fingertips. The faculty and instructors are there to help you. They are teaching you how to think like a nurse and how to apply the nursing process to patient care. Here are some examples of how this help can be provided.

" *Learning nursing is not like any other classes that students have taken before. Learning that they have to think differently and that they have to apply theoretical concepts to actual situations is difficult and new. Explaining why they have to know or do something a certain way doesn't make sense for beginning students. Providing rationales or explaining what can happen when you don't follow certain protocols or procedures seems to help them understand. Students should also seek advice when they don't understand concepts, when they are not doing well in classes, or are not performing well in clinical. If they can accept the advice and guidance and are willing to do things in a different way, slowly they learn to apply new thinking to their study strategies, to test-taking skills, and to their clinical practice.* "

—Edmonds, Washington; Nursing Instructor

" *I asked them for tips and hints on how to take exams, how to manage my time and handle patients, and I watched their example especially in terms of efficiency techniques and multitasking.* "

—Torrance, California; Nursing Student

"*Students need to keep an open mind as they approach new situations in the clinical arena. They need to correlate what they hear in the classroom with what they see with their patients, and the professor should be viewed as a tool to help the student make the necessary correlations and judgments. Professors are facilitators and guides for students, to help attain the goal of safe and informed practice. Students should read and question as much as they can and utilize the skills and support of their faculty to turn theory into practice. Students should never be afraid to ask questions about what they should do and should utilize the professor for feedback and encouragement throughout the process.*"

—**Union Beach, New Jersey;** Nursing Instructor

"*Students need instructors to provide emphasis and relevance. They often think every concept is important; yet we know some issues are more important than others. Without our insights into the importance and relevance, students can become lost without a strong foundation. I like a student who comes goal-directed, but for those that do not, I request appointments to create a direction for each of them. Strengths build out of weaknesses, yet each student will need our guidance.*"

—Phoenix, Arizona; Nursing Instructor

"*Ask your instructor what he or she would do in difficult situations so you can start critically thinking through situations. If you are unsure about something, ask your instructor for his or her opinion or where to go look for a solution.*"

—Mechanicsville, Maryland; Nursing Instructor

"*It has been my experience over the years I have taught nursing that the position of beginning students as just that, beginners, is very often not appreciated by faculty. Those who teach the initial nursing courses explain course policies and procedures, deliver content, and expect exam and clinical performance to be consistent with what would be expected of more advanced (farther along in their programs of study) students. Yes, it is true that nursing attracts many individuals who have already earned degrees in other areas or who have long been employed in other occupations, but anytime something new is being encountered, the learning curve is steep. Nursing students in beginning courses need to be taught how to study in a practice discipline. They need to understand that what is being learned is foundational to what will follow. Unlike what faculty often perceive, they do not intuitively know this.*

When given the tools of how to learn in nursing and other practice disciplines, students who are sincere in their desire to learn generally do well. Memorization is often sufficient in other non-nursing courses that they take, and they therefore attempt to use memorization as the learning approach in nursing. This does not usually serve them, since application and analysis are critical. Exercises in application of what they are being taught are essential for test success and for development of a usable body of knowledge."

—Southside, Alabama; Nursing Instructor

MAKE MAXIMUM USE OF THESE VALUABLE RESOURCES

In some classes you can sit in the back of the room, take notes, and passively absorb information needed for test taking. This is *not* the key to success in nursing school. Part of the assessment of your abilities will include your skills in communication and collaboration with your patients and with faculty and clinical staff members. You will be expected to contribute in clinical preconference and postconference. If you are unclear about what to contribute, you may begin by simply highlighting or summarizing the care and needs of your patient. Let the faculty members help you make the connection between what you are learning in the classroom and what you are experiencing in the practice setting.

"*Professors are your best advocates, but they can't advocate if they don't know what's going on.*"

—**San Jose, California;** Nursing Student

"*I see myself as a coach and mentor. I want students to 'bring something to the table.' By that I mean they should have something to contribute in the clinical setting—they should be prepared. I always tell them, 'You know more than you think you do.' I want them to pick my brain. Students should know the objectives of the clinical or classroom setting and make sure that I provide them with targeted learning experiences.*"

—**Old Bridge, New Jersey;** Nursing Instructor

"*Sometimes my clinical professor was more accessible than the nurse to whom I was assigned. It is always easier to do something correctly than it is to correct an error. I didn't hesitate to double-check with my clinical professor before I did anything that potentially could have injured my patient. Sometimes I just needed help (e.g., moving a patient who couldn't assist me with his or her own care). If another student nurse was not available, I would ask my clinical professor for assistance. I was never refused.*"

—**West Hartford, Connecticut;** Nursing Student

"*I relied on my instructors to answer any questions and as a sounding board when I was confused or uncertain. They are also a buffer if you have any problems with the health-care team where you are doing clinicals.*"

—**Manchester, Wisconsin;** Nursing Student

● *Don't assume we passed 'mind reading.' Approach us, ask your questions, tell us about your experiences, and help us learn what you specifically need.*

● *Make time to spend a few minutes with your clinical instructor each week, in his or her office. Use that time to clarify your understanding of assignments, concepts, instructions, test items, etc.*

● *Ask for patient assignments that 'match' the concepts or conditions that you are studying in class. Use that learning experience as an opportunity to apply what you are learning in class.*

● *Remember that knowing when to call for help is one of a nurse's greatest strengths. Your instructors value application of self-assessment skills.*

—**Fort Gibson, Oklahoma;** Nursing Instructor

"*The instructors are there to guide your learning experience—utilize this tool to the maximum potential. Don't be afraid to let the instructor know what you don't know. This is essential information for the instructor to know to best meet you where you are at. A good instructor will use this information to structure the clinical day accordingly.*"

—Madison, Indiana; Nursing Instructor

"*Students are not always sure why they are not succeeding academically or clinically. The process of discussing their concerns with professors is usually the best path for students to explore what could be obstacles to academic or clinical success. In the institutions in which I teach, we utilize a learning styles inventory to help students identify their learning strengths. This tool is often something advisors review with students to help them identify areas to focus on. There are also developmental issues with the student age group that just places them at risk for not utilizing the resources available to them.*"

—Philadelphia, Pennsylvania; Nursing Instructor

ASK AND ACT RESPONSIBLY AND PROFESSIONALLY

Your direct faculty member in the clinical setting may often be a different person than the classroom instructor. Hopefully, however, these faculty are coordinating and communicating so that your experience comes together as a whole. The faculty in both instances will expect that you show that you are motivated to become a successful professional nurse. In practical terms, this means coming to both class and clinical prepared. Both you and your submitted assignments need to be neat and professional. Take a look in the mirror before you rush off to clinical. Would you want the person who you see taking care of your mother? Although the faculty are there to help you, the relationship will work best if you remember to be polite, prepared, and respectful in your communication with them.

"*Think about the professors' schedules—the best time to approach is not just before class when they are setting up for class. Email them, use their office hours to make appointments, etc. Don't expect complicated questions to yield fast answers. Give professors time to answer an email or written request—no one is online 24/7! Do not make your emergency their emergency unless it is really warranted.*

Respectful communication is vital—use the names your professors have indicated they prefer. If they have given out their phone numbers, be judicious in using them. Make sure you have tried to find the answer to your question through rereading the syllabus or text or asking a classmate, before asking a professor if it pertains to course schedule or something clearly covered in the material. Profs appreciate students who have done the work before coming for help—don't come expecting a re-lecture! Make your questions specific. And THANK them for their help and advice. We don't need candy and flowers, but a simple thank-you and recognition that we gave up precious time to help is appreciated.

If you miss a class, make an effort to get the material from a classmate, then go over what is necessary with the professor; don't expect them to reteach it. Talk to professors about more than the class—they are people with lives and rich experiences. **"**

—Mishawaka, Indiana; Nursing Instructor

The education of nursing students is interactive, and you will form relationships with the nursing faculty. There will be instructors who you are drawn to as mentors and as human beings, while other faculty may not float your boat. You need to be open to learning from both types. Seek out time and support from those you are drawn to—they can become lifetime resources who can absolutely help you with your career over many years. Faculty get their professional reward from coaching and teaching bright, eager, motivated students. That means you!

CHAPTER 10

Taking Care of Yourself: Physically, Mentally, and Professionally

FINAL WORDS FROM INSTRUCTORS AND STUDENTS ON HOW NOT ONLY TO KEEP YOUR HEAD UP, BUT TO SUCCEED!

"*Knowledge, skills, energy, motivation—in two to three years, it happens.*"

—Amherst, Massachusetts; Nursing Student

The only resource that you truly are able to control is yourself and your well-being. We all have the same allotment of hours in a day, days in a week, and weeks in a year. School is a major commitment. By deciding to go to nursing school, you made the decision to put aside a number of things that you might not have time to do anymore. Sometimes this reality gets you down and you feel like the world is going by while you burn the midnight oil with studying, preparing for clinical, or doing an evening clinical rotation. A great deal of what you have to give as a nurse comes from way down inside yourself. Patients may be difficult, demanding, and physically and emotionally draining. To be able to go into clinical every day and give it your best, you need to take care of yourself—not only for your well-being, but also so that you can take care of your patients.

Taking care of yourself means getting enough sleep, eating a balanced diet, getting some exercise, enjoying time with your friends, and nurturing your spirit. Think of yourself as the instrument of patient care. Even a smart and competent nurse is less valuable if burned out or cranky. You may not experience such burnout as a student, but it is a common issue that many in the caring professions face when they avoid or neglect a planned approach to taking care of themselves. Unfortunately, many nurses have a track record of self neglect, martyrdom, and burnout. You can avoid this future by developing some self-care habits while you are a student.

"*Remember that the wonderful nurse who knows so much and seems so confident started out as a student not knowing anything.*"

—**La Porte, Texas;** Nursing Student

"*Stay away from negative thoughts and people. Exercise, eat properly, get enough sleep, and take care of your own health. Don't waste time on unimportant details. Deal with shortcomings head-on and seek out ways to improve skills.*"

—**Charlotte, North Carolina;** Nursing Instructor

"*Stay in the books. Don't get distracted. Dedicate yourself for the next two years and you'll be in command of a career where you decide where, what, when, and how much you work for. I don't know of any other career that offers those options.*"

—**Bayville, New Jersey;** Nursing Student

"*Be prepared and you'll make fewer mistakes. But take accountability for your actions. If something was not done correctly, learn from your mistake. And most important, have fun! Nursing is a great profession. You must enjoy what you do.*"

—**Charlotte, North Carolina; Nursing Instructor**

"*Gain the support of your family and friends. If you have friends or significant others who get in the way of studying, part from those relationships until you are through. Be true to yourself and your goals. Pray, have faith, and remember to laugh once in a while.*"

—**Floresville, Texas; Nursing Student**

"*Study hard and take your future profession seriously. It is not 'just a job,' so neither should nursing school be 'just school.' You will be responsible for human lives; use this time to come to terms with that and decide if it really is for you.*

Come up with a system that works for you—do you study best in the early morning or evening? Do you study best in a quiet library or noisy cafeteria? Are you an auditory (tape lectures) or visual (flashcards) learner? Use study groups. Take advantage of all the learning opportunities your clinicals provide: unit care conferences, committee meetings (you can sit in), MD rounds, etc. Ask experienced staff nurses if you can watch them do complicated dressing changes, listen to them do teaching, etc. "

—Rochester, Minnesota; Nursing Instructor

" *Nursing school becomes your life. You need to be willing to put your social life and recreational life on hold while you are in nursing school. You will not have time for both. You need to get involved in study groups, so that you can let your strengths benefit other students and you can benefit from their strengths. You need to have a support team—family, friends, other students, whomever—who will tell you when the stress is at its highest that this is all worth it and you are doing a great job.* "

—St. Charles, Illinois; Nursing Student

"*Expect to feel stressed and overwhelmed at times. There is a lot of information that you need to process in order to feel comfortable implementing it. That comfort does not come overnight, but rather with experience and an openness to asking 'why' questions.*"

—**New York, New York;** Nursing Instructor

"*If you find you don't like your first job, don't give up on nursing. You may simply not have found your niche within the profession.*"

—**Holt, Michigan;** Nursing Instructor

"*Start studying for the NCLEX as soon as you begin school because it is over before you know it. Don't be afraid to take on difficult patients and experiences because you feel uncomfortable—now is the time to learn before going out in the 'real world' without having an instructor right by your side the whole day.*"

—**Isanti, Minnesota;** Nursing Student

"*Stay focused, study hard, and keep all your notes from previous rotations accessible.*"

—Baltimore, Maryland; Nursing Student

"*Take the time and offer help to other students. Working as a cohesive group is vital to your success.*"

—North Aurora, Illinois; Nursing Student

"*Be an adult learner, and take responsibility for your education. Treat school like it is your job.*"

—Escondido, California; Nursing Instructor

"*Prioritize your assignments, work duties, and family stuff over and over until it works. It will also help you with prioritizing your patients' care.*"

—South St. Paul, Minnesota; Nursing Student

"*Ask questions and be involved. If you desire a specialty, ask to spend a day there. You are the one paying for your education—make the most of it.*"

—Eau Claire, Wisconsin; Nursing Student

"*Find your people. I feel that I had two girls who I always turned to when I needed something. Not all of your friends are going to know what it is like in nursing school. But my two girls were always there for me, when I wanted to cry about a clinical or had a question about a class.*"

—**Clinton, Iowa;** Nursing Student

"*Learn as much as you can but also know that the learning does not stop when you leave your last class—it's a lifelong process.*"

—**Norfolk, Nebraska;** Nursing Student

"*Find out what your learning style is and figure out how to use it to your success. Use your resources: your instructors, the lab, the library, etc. Learn all that you can and take one day at a time. Don't ever put yourself down and don't compare yourself to others. I always did that and it made me stress more. Do the best that YOU can do!*"

—**Lancaster, California;** Nursing Student

"*It's a long haul but worth it in the end! Keep reading, studying, and laughing.*"

—**Mendota, Illinois;** Nursing Student

"*Cut out distractions that take your attention away from your goals. Make your personal success your priority! No one else is going to look out for you but you.*"

—**Houston, Texas;** Nursing Student

"*Take each day at a time and don't freak out with each new thing. You* will *learn it and it's not as difficult as it may seem at first. It takes time to learn things, and you have plenty of time to do it in.*"

—**Mesa, Arizona;** Nursing Student

"*Be positive. You were smart enough to get* in *to nursing school; determination will get you* through *it. Avoid the whining and complaining that some people fall into; it doesn't help anyone. There will always be tough teachers and bad test questions—let it go. Smile, relax, and breathe. When you need a break, go for a long walk and smile!"*

—Boston, Massachusetts; Nursing Student

"Support one another. Nursing students understand each other and the multiple stresses involved in nursing school."

—Holt, Michigan; Nursing Instructor

"Don't cram for an exam, keep up with the reading . . . not just to pass the exam, but for your future. It's not about getting good grades; this is your foundation for your future practice. Don't shoot yourself in the foot. Make sure you are getting the most out your education—your practice depends on it!"

—Albuquerque, New Mexico; Nursing Student

"Get excited about clinical. You can learn so much in eight hours."

—Madison, Wisconsin; Nursing Student

"*Ask questions constantly. Never be satisfied with an answer you don't understand. Trust your gut. If it doesn't seem right, double-check and find out why.*"

—Abilene, Texas; Nursing Student

"*Balance is the key. You must find a balance between school, work, family, and 'me' time.*"

—Pasadena, California; Nursing Student

"*Listen very carefully. If you are unclear on anything, ask questions. Never assume. If you have worked in the health-care field before going to nursing school, remember that things are not done the same way in school as they are done in the real world, so do as you are told! Stay on top of things, and if there are areas you don't understand—such as fluids and electrolytes or the endocrine system or anything for that matter—get help early. These are things you will need throughout your entire time in nursing school. They can come back again and again to haunt you. And all the systems work together, so if you have a hard time with one, others will suffer too.*"

—Monona, Iowa; Nursing Student

"*Invest in the experience as completely as possible. Accept limitations for the period of time necessary to be successful in nursing school and for yourself.*"

   —Brookeland, Texas; Nursing Instructor

"*Do lots, lots, lots of study groups if you can and if that is what works for you. Talk about your anxiety and fears with other students or instructors. I believe it helps you work through those fears and you realize you are not the only one. Study, study, study, and buy a NCLEX review book early—don't wait until after school is done to start looking at NCLEX-style questions. I bought mine during my third semester and skimmed it every night, and I believe that helped prepare me.*"

   —Tucson, Arizona; Nursing Student

"*Get the most out of clinical time that you can— volunteer to stay extra hours, do procedures for as many nurses as will let you, and practice, practice, practice. When you graduate it is so different than clinical, because you are now ultimately responsible for your actions. What a great feeling to have.*"

—Corpus Christi, Texas; Nursing Student

"*The best way to survive nursing school is to believe in yourself. If you don't believe you can pass a course or succeed in clinical, you never will. Always strive to be the best and know what you are doing. If you have a question, ask. That is why your clinical instructors are there. Last, study as much as possible. There is no way you can pass nursing school just by sliding by.*"

—Yutan, Nebraska; Nursing Student

"*Be prepared to be tired, but happy.*"

—Noble, Oklahoma; Nursing Student

"*Get plenty of rest and learn to listen to your body. Your body will tell you when enough is enough. Sometimes you just need to call it a day and go to bed or get a nap.*"

—Hanover, Pennsylvania; Nursing Student

"*Do your best to stay ahead of the game; however, know that you will never feel that you are caught up. Be okay with that.*"

—**McHenry, Illinois;** Nursing Student

"*Evaluate your life, and learn to say NO while you are in nursing school. Plan a reward at the end of each semester or year. Enlist family members to help you with things like laundry. Keep your long-term goal in mind. It is always going to take more effort than you imagine, so simplify your life in as many ways as possible prior to starting nursing school. If you have a family, consider spacing out your program over several years to decrease the stress. Learn to laugh.*"

—**Mishawaka, Indiana;** Nursing Instructor

"*Have a countdown calendar so you know how much longer you have, and cross each week off as you go. This is a visual encouragement in the middle when time seems so slow. I started with 68 weeks, and each month I watched as that number grew smaller. I was excited for the numbers to be under 52, 25, 10, then 9 . . . 8 . . . 7 . . . 6 . . . 5 . . . 4 . . . 3 . . . 2 . . . 1. WOW, that was good for me and also my children to see go by! Also, have a special something at the end of each nursing block,* like a *big dinner or even a weekend trip.*"

—**Mesa, Arizona;** Nursing Student

"*Do your very best and give a 100 percent honest effort to strive for your dreams. It took my whole family to help me make it through nursing school—my husband, kids, parents—everybody pitched in somewhere along the line just so I could finish.*"

—**Pittsburgh, Pennsylvania;** Nursing Student

"*Remember that school is temporary—but remind your friends that school comes first for now and that you will be able to see them more after your schooling is finished.*"

—**Lincoln, Nebraska;** Nursing Instructor

> "*Recognize that most of this will be a new experience. Stay on your toes but enjoy the journey. Handle situations that come up quickly so you can keep stress to a minimum. Learn to love what you are doing.*"
>
> —**Centennial, Colorado;** Nursing Instructor

Throughout this book many of the experts—both students and faculty—have pointed out that nursing can be challenging work. It is stressful, sometimes physically challenging, and often filled with intense emotions. You will be able to function most effectively if you start from the beginning with good self-care habits. You may be asked to rotate shifts between evenings, nights, or days. Many nurses currently work 12-hour shifts or are asked to work overtime or extra duty. You need to establish your own plan for survival and self-care to meet challenges like these, and others.

Having balance between your career as a nurse and your personal life is important. Try your best not to take your work home with you in your head or your heart. A tip to accomplish this is to plan a transition activity after work. Come home, take a hot shower, change into your comfortable clothing, ride your bike, go work out at the gym, or listen to some soothing music. Avoid calling up another nurse or coworker and rehashing the day. You need a break from your nurse role. For those of you with young children, this transition time may be more difficult to arrange, but try if you can to do something fun and enjoy your time with the kids. Spend some time finding out what activities and actions from others make *you* feel cared for. You will have more to give to others if you are on the receiving end of some nurturing yourself.

Final Words

Just the fact that you went out of your way to get this book is a sign that you are a committed nursing student. You are seeking ideas and suggestions to be the best that you can be as a student and future nurse. Good for you and way to go! Half of being successful is showing up and being ready to go the extra mile. I worked for a great nursing leader who was consistently 30 minutes early for all of her appointments. She spent her time on the way home from off-site meetings sending thank-you notes to the people she just met with. It works. Try a bit harder and your effort will pay off for you and for your patients.

Let's review some of the key takeaway ideas from this book:

- Being a new student in a clinical setting is going to be a challenge.
- You need to be as prepared as you can before you go to clinical.

- Find out as much as you can in advance about your patient, and study up on his or her diagnosis, medications, and care needs.

- Apply the nursing process, which is also the scientific process. Collect data, analyze the information you have observed, provide interventions, and then evaluate the impact of the interventions on the patient, and their outcomes.

- Patients are grateful for your care, even if they can't express themselves—they may be grumpy or difficult, but remember they are sick and you are not. Thinking this way can make a lot of difference. Do not take unpleasant behaviors personally.

- Some patients will steal your heart and others will be difficult. Get ready for both types and many in between.

- Go out of your way to learn all you can. Ask to go observe diagnostic tests and procedures, help your fellow students, and talk with your patients when you have a chance.

- Learn what you can from experienced staff nurses and faculty. Settings that take on students do so because they believe strongly that everyone benefits from having students on-site. Take advantage of this experience and get the most you can from it.

- Don't be afraid to ask questions and seek guidance. You are in the learning mode and this is how you will learn. Try to find faculty members who care and who relate to you, and seek them out.

- Learn how to document carefully and effectively in patients' charts. The documentation should be descriptive and factual without being ponderous.

- Take care of yourself. Expect the nursing program and the clinical to be a taxing effort. Make time for school to be a major priority in your life.

I have had the pleasure of being a nurse for about 30 years. I have not regretted this career choice for one moment. Thinking back to my clinical experiences as a student, my chief memories are of feeling awkward, not knowing what to do, whom to talk to, or how to act. In the psych ward, my fellow students and I were so afraid of the patients that we walked around like a gaggle of geese. I remember the day one of my friends gave her postoperative patient double the dose of morphine that was ordered! She also asked a quadriplegic patient if he felt like a head lying on the pillow. It made me crazy that the only people who were up to ever eat breakfast at our dorm were the nursing students. But obviously, I survived and I thrived. Thirty years later, I have the joy and the formidable responsibility of working with both undergraduate and graduate student nurses. I can safely say that nothing has been more rewarding to me in my career. I wish you the very best in the important work you are doing. You will change lives.

OWENS COMMUNITY COLLEGE
P.O. Box 10,000
Toledo, OH 43699-1947